Diffusion Tensor Imaging and Fractional Anisotropy

Rahul P. Kotian • Prakashini Koteshwar

Diffusion Tensor Imaging and Fractional Anisotropy

Imaging Biomarkers in Early Parkinson's Disease

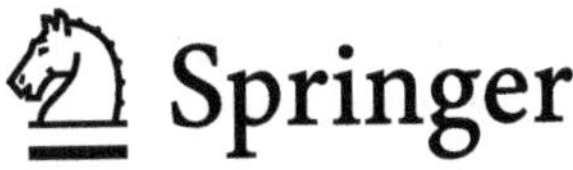

Rahul P. Kotian
Department of Anatomy
Saveetha Dental College
Saveetha Institute of Medical & Technical Sciences
Chennai, Tamil Nadu, India

Prakashini Koteshwar
Department of Radio-Diagnosis & Imaging
Kasturba Medical College
Manipal Academy of Higher Education
Manipal, Karnataka, India

ISBN 978-981-19-5003-2 ISBN 978-981-19-5001-8 (eBook)
https://doi.org/10.1007/978-981-19-5001-8

This Springer imprint is published by the registered company Springer Nature Singapore Pte Ltd.
The registered company address is: 152 Beach Road, #21-01/04 Gateway East, Singapore 189721, Singapore

"There is no end to education. It is not that you read a book, pass an examination, and finish your education. Your entire life, from the moment you are born to the moment you die, is a process of learning".

This book is dedicated with love and affection to my beautiful, smart and overall cute and witty wife ***Disha R. Kotian.*** *You bring so much joy and happiness to my life.*

This book is also dedicated to my loving ***Father, Pratap N. Kotian****, who is truly the unsung hero of my life and whose unceasing efforts and sacrifices have made me who I am today.*

The important people in our lives have left imprints. They may stay or go in the physical world, but they always remain in our hearts forever, because they have helped us from the bottom of their heart. And, there's no getting over that.

I also dedicate this book to my little sister, Dr. ***Sneha P. Kotian,*** *my late* ***Mother Uma P. Kotian****, my greatest late grandfather* ***Shambhu K. Jathan*** *and lastly my dearest late Dr.* ***Smiti S****. A special mention and* *thanks to my loving in-laws* ***Mr. Mohan Singh Faujdar*** *and* ***Mrs. Vinita Singh*** *for their unconditional love and support.*

"Cricket is not everything, not by any means, but it has been a very large part of whom I am today! Self-confidence has always been one of my good qualities. I am always very confident. It is in my nature to be confident and to be aggressive. And it applies in my batting, fielding, and bowling".

Foreword

Diffusion Tensor Imaging and Fractional Anisotropy: Imaging Biomarkers in Early Parkinson's Disease—A comprehensive textbook for undergraduate, postgraduate and doctoral medical imaging technology students is a complete package for comprehending the complex physics of DTI and its clinical correlation to Parkinson's disease. Magnetic resonance imaging (MRI) has advanced dramatically as a clinical tool, far outpacing the rate of development of any other imaging technique. Medical imaging specialists have historically been slow to grasp the physics of MRI and apply it in clinical practice. The underlying technology in MRI is complex and having a working understanding of it is critical for good clinical practice. As a result, the radiologist requires the assistance of imaging technologists who are not only capable but also well informed to a degree not required in other radiological work. Without a doubt, MRI is the modality where the changing dynamics of technology and applications pose the greatest challenges for continuing education.

This book's success should come as no surprise given the need for it and the fact that it was written by an imaging technologist/radiographer (Dr. Rahul Pratap Kotian) and a radiologist (Dr. Prakashini K.), both of whom are actively involved in MRI, not only in clinical imaging but also in academic teaching to other aspiring students. I enthusiastically support this new initiative of writing a comprehensive textbook on DTI, and I am confident that it will be useful to readers in the field of medical imaging technology.

Manipal Academy of Higher Education
Manipal, Karnataka, India

H. S. Ballal

Preface

My journey in the Medical Imaging field transformed me into an academician and researcher. This transformation was always fuelled by the ulterior motive to serve the community and the nation at large. I was particularly attracted to Magnetic Resonance Imaging (MRI) in the year 2005, not due to its magnetic properties but a rather unfortunate incident at my mother's MRI scan. I was amazed and curious at the same time to see how the MRI scan could miraculously detect my mother's ailments within a short span of 45 min of scanning.

At that very moment, I decided to pursue a career in MRI and during my entire undergraduate and postgraduate study duration I focused on learning the basics and advancements in the field of MRI with the kind help and support of some fabulous Radiologists at Kasturba Medical College, Department of Radiology, MAHE, Manipal. The idea of writing a book on Diffusion Tensor Imaging (DTI) and Fractional Anisotropy (FA) in Early Parkinson's disease was developed during my PhD study in 2017 where I was working on one of my publications related to FA and DTI and realized its growing need and applications in clinical imaging, diagnosis and treatment. There was clearly a gap in the literature regarding the understanding of these newly developed advanced imaging techniques in MRI, namely DTI and FA.

This book would be a classical fit for both the medical imaging technologist and radiologist as it gives a brief overview of MRI-DTI and FA-related physics, protocols, instrumentation and key clinical imaging biomarker findings in early Parkinson's disease. All of the information in this book is unique, based on my extensive knowledge of DTI, FA, and Parkinson's disease, which I gained throughout my PhD research among the Indian people. Parkinson's disease has not been taken seriously in India until recently, and my research findings are a small attempt to help the people of my nation. I am convinced that assisting in the early detection of even one Parkinson's disease case using the knowledge offered in this book would make our research work invaluable.

A glossary of common terms and appendices on acronyms are also included. I believe that this book fulfils its purpose and will support the education of Radiographers, Medical Imaging Technologists and Radiologists in the glorious art and science of MRI.

I am particularly grateful and honoured to learn and work with the following people in my medical imaging career: Dr. H. S. Ballal (Pro-Chancellor, Manipal) Dr. Prakashini K. (PhD guide), Dr. N. Sreekumaran Nair (PhD co-guide), Dr. Satish

M. Babu (PhD co-guide), Dr. Goutham Kumar Puppala (Neurologist), Dr. B. Rajashekhar (Dynamic Allied Health Dean), Dr. G. Arun Maiya (Dean Allied Health), Dr. Animesh Hazari (Strong influencer for my book write-up), Adithya G. Rao (Book diagram editing), Disha Kotian (Book diagram and general editing), Mr. P. N. Joshi (First Medical Imaging Teacher), Mr. Barty Vinod (Teacher), Ms. Nilna Narayanan (Teacher), Mr. Sushil Yadav (Teacher), Dr. Suresh Sukumar (Teacher), Dr. V. R. K. Rao (Radiologist), Dr. Rajgopal K. V. (Radiologist), Dr. Puneet (Radiologist), Dr. Sonali Ullal (Radiologist), Dr. Anand Venugopal (Radiologist), Dr. Chandrakant Shetty (Radiologist), Dr. Samir (Radiologist), Dr. Laxmikanth (Radiologist), Dr. Naveen Mulimani (Radiologist), Dr. Mohammad Rawashdeh (Mentor), Dr. Saikiran (Colleague), Dr. Winniecia (Colleague), Mr. Sharath (Colleague), Mr. Ren Trevor (Friend), Dr. Dhanashekhar (mentor and close friend), Dr. Fiddy Davis (mentor and close friend), Dr. Raghu (Mentor and close friend), Dr. Kishan (Mentor and close friend), Mr. Vivek (Mentor and close friend), Dr. Sentil (Senior), Dr. Gopi (Senior Teacher and Research Co-ordinator), Dr. Hari (Mentor) and Dr. John Solomon (Research Co-ordinator).

A very special thanks to all my technical medical imaging staff at Kasturba Hospital, Manipal from whom I learned the art of MRI patient scanning: Joshi sir, Prakash Sir, Satish sir, Sumana madam, Vidya Madam, Amitha Madam and all senior members of the team.

I also thank Dr. Pradeep Goud (Vice-Chancellor) and Dr. Lavanya (Professor) for my current affiliations and long-term research associations.

Lastly, I am very grateful to all the Universities which I was associated with in my entire medical imaging career, namely Manipal College of Health Professions, Manipal Academy of Higher Education, Kasturba Medical College, Srinivas University, NIMS University, Assam Downtown University, Gulf Medical University, SRI Devraj URS Academy of Higher Education and Research, Saveetha Dental College, Saveetha Institute of Medical and Technical Sciences, Goa Medical College, NITTE Educational Trust, TCS iON, Tata Consultancy Services and Shri Jagdishprasad Jhabarmal Tibrewala University.

Last but not least, I humbly thank all my Radiography Professional body affiliations.

- Indian Society of Radiological Technologists (ISRT), India
- Radiological Society of North America (RSNA)
- European Society of Radiology (ESR), Europe
- International Society of Radiographers and Radiological Technologists (ISRRT)
- Karnataka Medical Radiographers and Allied Technologists Association, India
- Indian Association of Radiological Technologists (IART), India
- Global Illuminators, Kuala Lumpur, Malaysia

Chennai, Tamil Nadu, India Rahul P. Kotian

Preface

This small but well-organized and focused book is an educational achievement in the field of Diffusion Tensor Imaging of the Brain. It is well established that the DTI plays an important role in both pre-op and post-op evaluation of brain tumours. However, without understanding the physics and principles of DTI, it is difficult to comprehend. With this goal in mind, we compiled a small compilation of everything about DTI in the brain. The chapters are written in the order of simple to complex topics, and they cover many relevant previous several year reviews and Scrivener's thoughts.

This compilation is the result of my mentorship on the topic of "DTI in normal white matter and diffuse brain diseases". Back in 2012, it was thought to be difficult to learn DTI principles.

Manipal, Karnataka, India — Prakashini Koteshwar

Contents

About the Authors

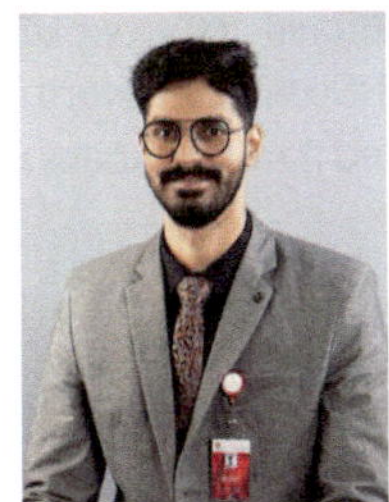

Dr Rahul P. Kotian, PhD - MRI is currently working at the Department of Anatomy as an Adjunct Professor, at Saveetha Dental College, Saveetha Institute of Medical & Technical Sciences, Chennai, India. Dr. Rahul is also working as a Visiting Professor at SRI Devraj URS Academy of Higher Education & Research, Kolar, Karnataka India. Dr Rahul is also currently serving as an Expert Panel in Medical Imaging Technology at TCS iON, Tata Consultancy Services, India. Dr Rahul was also part of the Medical Imaging Sciences Program at the College of Health Sciences, Gulf Medical University, Ajman, the United Arab Emirates from September 2021 – September 2022 and has teaching and research experience of 13 years in the field of Medical Imaging. Dr Rahul also served at Manipal College of Health Professions, and Manipal Academy of Higher Education for over a decade in different capacities from 2009-to 2019. Dr Rahal was also the former Dean & Professor at the College of Allied Health Sciences, NIMS University, Jaipur, Rajasthan. Dr Rahul was also the Associate Dean, Professor & Head of Medical Imaging at the College of Allied Health Sciences, Srinivas University, Mukka, Mangalore, Karnataka, India. Dr Rahul P Kotian is a Magnetic Resonance Imaging doctorate and received his PhD from Manipal College of Health Professions, Manipal Academy of Higher Education, Manipal, Karnataka, India. During this study tenure, he was awarded as the best outgoing student at the graduate (B.Sc. Medical Imaging Technology, 2009) and post-graduate (M.Sc. Medical Imaging Technology, 2011) levels. Dr Rahul was also the first Clinical PhD in Magnetic Resonance Imaging and Parkinson's disease in Medical Imaging in India. Dr Rahul P Kotian was also recognized with Honorary Doctorate for his excellence in the field of Medical Imaging Technology on 12th September 2021 from Bharat Virtual University for Peace and Education (Unit of United Nations Organization, Geneva). He has published several scientific research papers in the field of Medical Imaging, Radiology and

Magnetic Resonance Imaging (MRI), Diffusion Tensor Imaging (DTI), Fractional Anisotropy (FA), Parkinson's disease (PD), Computed Tomography (CT) and Radiation Protection and contributed extensively to the medical imaging literature. He is an active member as a Reviewer for many Scopus-indexed peer-reviewed journals. He was also the Radiation Safety officer Level I officer at Kasturba Medical College and Hospital, Manipal Academy of Higher Education. (2011–2014, 2014–2017 and 2017–2019). He is recognized internationally and nationally as a leader in the field of Medical Imaging in DTI and FA imaging and has presented several research papers. He is also one of the keynote and guest speakers at various International (European Congress of Radiology – Austria, Radiological Society of North America and Annual Radiology meet – the United Arab Emirates) and National Conferences.

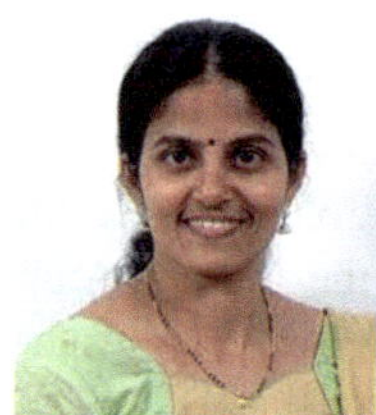

Dr Prakashini Koteshwar, MD Radio-Diagnosis is a Professor in the Department of Radiology, Kasturba Medical College, Manipal Academy of Higher Education, Manipal, Udupi, Karnataka, and serving at Kasturba Medical college since 2006. She perused her MD degree in Radiodiagnosis and Imaging from a prestigious university, KMC, Manipal Academy of Higher Education.

Since then, she is serving at her alma mater at different cadre, and since 2014 she is positioned as a Professor. She is currently heading the Department of Radiology at Kasturba Medical College since 2018. During her tenure, she initiated different academic programmes and recently commenced the Interventional Division which is going to provide all high-end semi-invasive non-surgical options of treatment, to various emergency and non-emergency conditions.

Her area of interest is Neuroimaging, Cardiovascular Imaging and Interventional Radiology. She has completed Level I accreditation in CT and MRI reporting of Cardiac Imaging. She has been working with AI-based algorithm applications in brain tumours and computational flow dynamics in carotid, renal arteries and presently on "the effect of peristalsis on ureteric flow".

She has several publications into her credit both in National and International reputed journals on clinical, radiological and AI aspects. She has been guiding several research and PhD projects of MD Radiology, MSc Medical Imaging students and also engineering graduates.

She is an auditor of NABH, ISO accreditation and in charge of the documents related to MCI recognition for MBBS and MD radiology. She is also currently working with grant projects of DST/SERB and industry collaborations too.

List of Figures

List of Tables

1 History and Basic Principles of Magnetic Resonance Imaging

The foundation of learning magnetic resonance imaging (MRI) lies behind understanding the basic principles of hydrogen nuclei and their associated spin within the human body. It is therefore very vital to understand these basics before discussing complex areas in MRI. This chapter throws light on some of the key inventions in the field of magnetic resonance imaging. A brief explanation about the basic principles involved in MRI along with its associated software and hardware is highlighted.

1.1 Introduction to MRI

Magnetic resonance imaging (MRI) is a non-ionizing imaging technique that has been utilized in clinical medicine for over 50 years. When compared to other medical imaging modalities that use ionizing radiation, such as computed tomography (CT), conventional angiography, fluoroscopy and conventional radiography, this imaging modality provides excellent soft-tissue imaging with contrast resolution in various parts of the body such as the brain grey and white matter, muscles, ligaments, blood flow and so on. The most significant advantage of MRI over other imaging modalities is that it uses strong magnetic field strengths for imaging, as opposed to other modalities that use ionizing radiation such as X-rays. MRI produces multiplanar views of the human body by using hydrogen nuclei that are abundant in the human body, whereas X-rays interact directly with the patient's body and then produce images of the internal organs of the body via ionization.

R. P. Kotian, P. Koteshwar, *Diffusion Tensor Imaging and Fractional Anisotropy*,
https://doi.org/10.1007/978-981-19-5001-8_1

1.2 History and Roadmap to Innovations in MRI

Going way back to the year 1827, when the utility of MRI was not sensed, the random continuous motion of pollen grains suspended in water was studied by Sir Robert Brown using a microscope. Thereafter, the name Brownian motion was bestowed in his honour. The water molecules can move in all directions in pure water, without any restrictions, i.e. it demonstrates isotropic diffusion. This diffusion of water molecules in the water medium is referred to as self-diffusion. The diffusion coefficient can be calculated using particle/molecule size, solvent/fluid medium viscosity and temperature. The distance covered by water molecules over time represents the unrestricted isotropic diffusion of water molecules in a specified direction. The water molecule diffusion coefficient is directly proportional to temperature and rises by 2.4% per 1 °C. At 25 °C, the diffusion coefficient of water molecules is 2.3×10^{-3} mm^2/s, and at body temperature (37 °C), it is 3×10^{-3} mm^2/s [1, 2].

The basic idea behind MRI is that strong magnetic fields are used to excite specific atoms within the body, and then radiofrequency pulses are used to change their alignment. Carr, the legendary MRI researcher, published a paper on the effects of diffusion on free precession in 1954. In 1950, he went to Sir Erwin Hahn's laboratory and discovered that Hahn used equal pulses with spin echo to investigate depth in diffusion imaging. Carr expanded on this technique by correcting signal decay by diffusion with a 90° pulse followed by several 180° pulses (Carr-Purcell theory). The results showed that the transverse decay accurately represented the T2 relaxation times of the spins [3]. In 1968, Tanner and Stejskal released a paper on diffusion describing their fresh modified spin-echo method "pulsed-gradient" and then using the method used by Hahn, Carr and Purcell to measure diffusion [3, 4]. Many research studies have been published for limited diffusion, including minute cavities and small regions between parallel barriers. They discovered an association in the kinetics of diffusion between limited diffusion and tissue composition. In the 1970s, Peter Mansfield developed a technique for rapid imaging (30–100 ms) known as echo-planar imaging (EPI), which is commonly used in modern diffusion-weighted imaging (DWI). In the early 1980s, diffusion was regarded as the normal gold diagnostic instrument for neurological disorders. A well-known scientist named Bihan later outlined the use of the "microscopic random translation movement" of fluid molecules to acquire significant tissue physiological information. Diffusion causes random dephasing and thus attenuates voxel signal. This impact can be captured and visualized using a coefficient of diffusion that can be calculated using gradient-echo pulses [5].

Magnetic resonance phenomenon was discovered way back in the year 1946, and even after this invention, only spectroscopic analysis of samples was possible, until Sir Paul Lauterbur and Sir Peter Mansfield introduced magnetic field gradients and Fourier transform for image reconstruction [6]. It was during the same time where we saw Sir Felix Bloch and Sir Edward Purcell discovering the nuclear magnetic resonance phenomena independently for which they won the Nobel Prize in 1952. Later based on these research findings in 1977, the legends Sir Damadian, Sir

Minkoff and Sir M. Goldsmith performed the first MRI scan of a human being [7]. These scientists created MRI into a revolutionary technology with the advent of EPI, which was a fast-imaging technique by Sir Mansfield in 1977. Sir Michael Moseley published a paper in 1990 on the early detection of regional cerebral ischemia in cats, which was supplemented with routine MRI, DWI and magnetic resonance spectroscopy (T2-weighted). The findings of the research showed that DWI was very helpful and appropriate for detecting ischemic impacts [8]. After occlusion of middle cerebral and carotid arteries of cats, they identified regions of ischemic injury in only 45 min strongly using diffusion-weighted sequences. Meanwhile, the T2-weighted spin-echo images were unable to demonstrate brain injury within 2–3 h as it takes time to show any significant changes. In 1990, Sir Moseley released another paper describing a method for detecting anisotropic water diffusion in a cat's central nervous system using DWI and proposed that this method could be used in brain and spinal cord assessment of white-matter tracts. As expected, a unique DWI application called diffusion-tensor imaging (DTI) was then discovered that could image the brain's white-matter tracts [9].

The advent of superconducting magnets is still considered MRI's most pioneering innovation, which made it possible to use powerful magnetic fields in the imaging [10]. Since then, faster imaging techniques with echo-planar and parallel imaging techniques have made MRI one of the best imaging modalities. The reconstruction mathematics utilized in MRI was developed by Sir Peter Mansfield, who soon developed EPI which produced images in seconds, and now this technique is used on all current scanners. The new era of imaging began in the late 1990s and early 2000s when we saw cardiac, body, fetal and functional MRI growing and developing rapidly. Revolutionary advances in the field of MRI were seen in 2003 when Sir Paul C. Lauterbur and Peter Mansfield received the Noble Award for their discovery of using MRI as a diagnostic imaging instrument [11–16].

MRI is a versatile imaging modality known for its diverse image contrast techniques that employ several sequences to produce T1, T2, T2* and proton density-weighted images. The widespread use of contrast agents based on MR gadolinium has resulted in its widespread use.

1.3 Atomic Structure

An atom is the tiniest component of an element. It is made up of protons, neutrons and electrons. Protons are positively charged particles that are found in the nucleus. Electrons are negatively charged and they revolve around the nucleus in specific shells. However, the neutrons have no charge and are situated at the nucleus of the atom. The structure and motion of atoms are very well depicted in Fig. 1.1. The total number of protons in the nucleus is defined as the atomic number. The mass number is defined as the sum of the nucleus's protons and neutrons. Finally, isotopes are atoms of the same element with different mass numbers.

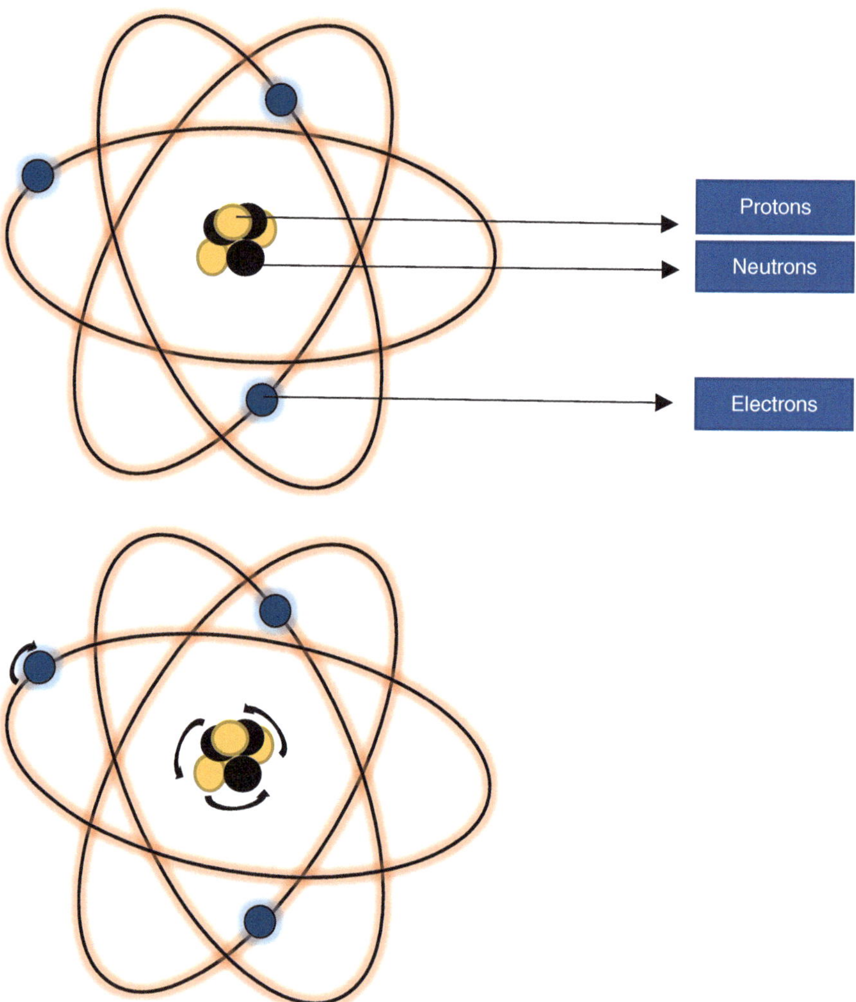

Fig. 1.1 Structure and motion of particles in an atom

1.3.1 Motion Within the Atom

The motion within the atom forms the basis of magnetic resonance imaging. The electrons are negatively charged spin on their axis and also revolve around the nucleus in different shell orbits. The nucleus revolves around its axis. The atom's typical motion and spin generate a magnetic field around it, which serves as the foundation for magnetic resonance imaging [17].

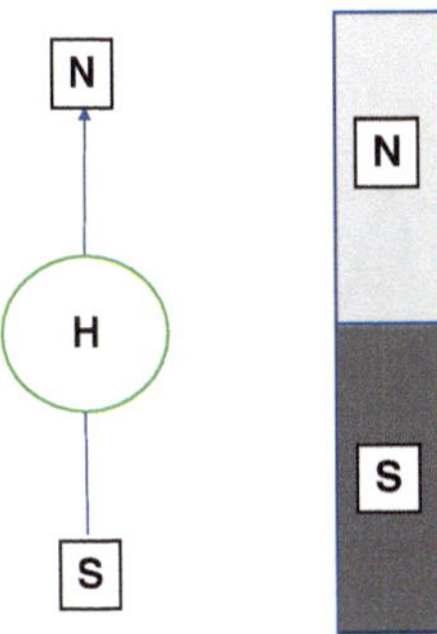

Fig. 1.2 Hydrogen nucleus with its magnetic moment

1.3.2 Hydrogen as MR Active Nucleus

MR active nucleus with a single solitary proton and odd mass number is characterized by its unique property of aligning itself to an applied external magnetic field. The MR active nucleus employed in clinical MRI is the hydrogen nucleus. The large abundance of hydrogen nuclei within the human body along with its single solitary proton makes it the best fit for MRI. The hydrogen proton possesses both the net charge and net spin. A magnetic field is created around the hydrogen nucleus as a result of this property. Figure 1.2 depicts an arrow indicating the size and direction of this magnetic field. The arrow direction denotes the magnetic moment's alignment direction, whereas the length denotes the magnetic moment's magnitude [18].

1.4 Alignment and Precession

1.4.1 Alignment

The alignment process by the MR active nucleus can be described using both classical and quantum theory. The MR active nucleus will take any random direction and orientation in the absence of an external magnetic field. When a magnetic field is applied from outside, the MR active nucleus aligns itself in the direction of the main magnetic field. This is referred to as alignment, and it is depicted in Fig. 1.3. Figure 1.4 depicts how the classical theory explains the direction of magnetic moments using parallel and antiparallel alignment. Magnetic moments align themselves in the direction of the main magnetic field in parallel alignment, whereas magnetic moments align themselves in the opposite direction of the main magnetic field in antiparallel alignment. The net magnetization vector (NMV) always aligns itself to the direction of the main magnetic field (parallel alignment) at room temperature (thermal equilibrium).

Quantum theory explains alignment using spin-up (parallel direction) and spin-down (antiparallel direction) nuclei by focusing on the energy level of the nuclei. The magnetic field strength (B_0), measured in tesla, is another factor that influences nuclei alignment. The theory further states that in the presence of an external

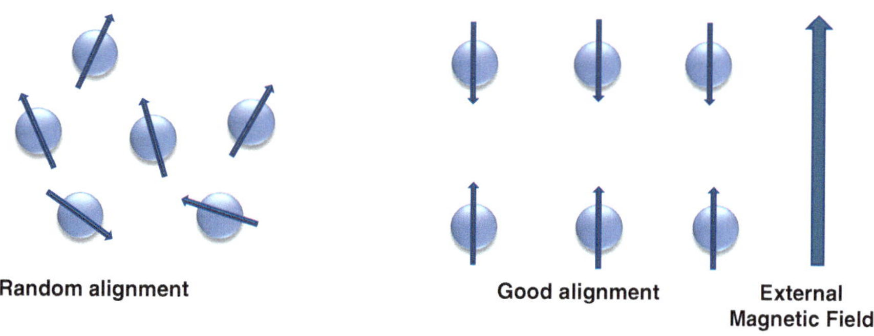

Fig. 1.3 Effects of magnetic field on MR active nucleus

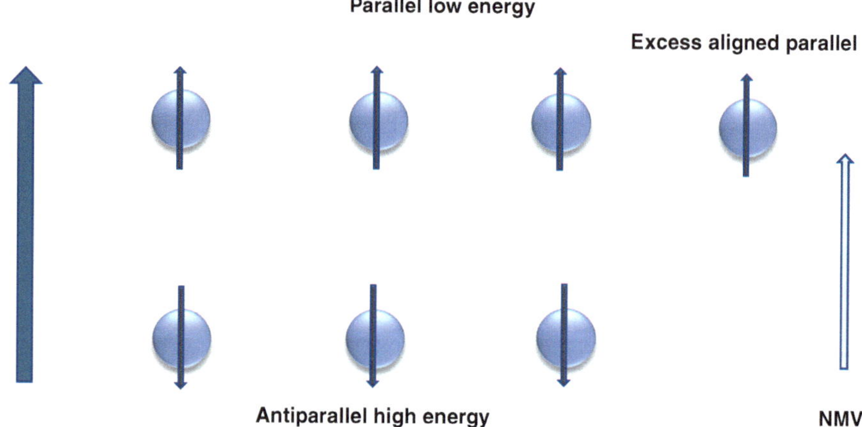

Fig. 1.4 Classical theory alignment

magnetic field, the hydrogen nuclei also called the MR active nucleus align either in the spin-up or spin-down direction. The majority of the nuclei possess low energy and hence align parallel to the main magnetic field. However, a small portion of the nuclei possesses enough energy to oppose the main magnetic field and hence align antiparallel to it.

Both theories discussed above can be correlated to the clinical MR imaging scenario where we deal with patients. The patient's body temperature plays an important role in imaging to determine whether the nucleus is in low or high energy states. In routine clinical imaging, we assume the patient's temperature to be constant and not fluctuate much. As the magnitude of the external magnetic field increases, the majority of the magnetic moments of the nuclei line up in the parallel direction. In contrast to the antiparallel direction, the low energy population grows as the field strength grows. As a result, the net magnetization vector expands (NMV) [18–21] (Fig. 1.5).

1.4.2 Precession

The MR active nucleus, as discussed in the previous subsection of this chapter, is constantly spinning around its axis. The external magnetic field's effect on the MR active nuclei induces a secondary spin known as spin wobble, and this process is known as wobbling. This wobbling phenomenon as well as the circular path followed by MR active nuclei around the external magnetic field (B_0) is called precession as depicted in Fig. 1.6. The speed at which this wobbling phenomenon occurs is called the precessional frequency.

In a given magnetic field, the Larmor equation can be used to calculate the frequency and speed of precession for an MR active nucleus. The following formulas can be used to calculate the Larmor equation:

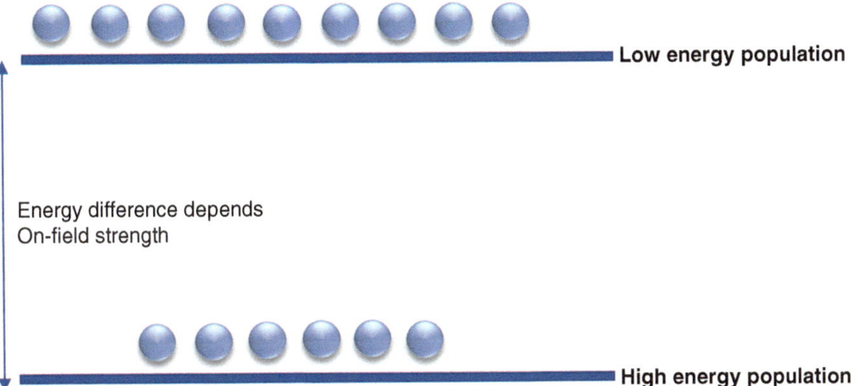

Fig. 1.5 Quantum theory alignment

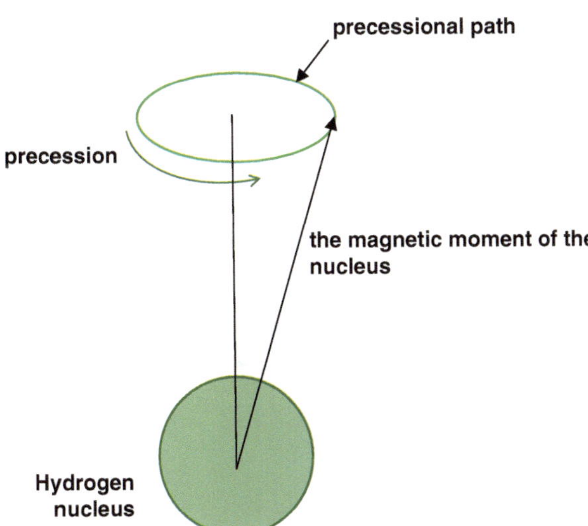

Fig. 1.6 MR active nuclei precession and wobbling phenomenon

$$\omega_0 = B_0 \times \lambda$$

where

ω_0 = precessional frequency of MR active hydrogen nuclei
B_0 = strength of the external magnetic field
λ = gyromagnetic ratio

The gyromagnetic ratio is defined as the precessional frequency of a specific nucleus at 1 T and is measured in MHz/T units. The gyromagnetic ratio of hydrogen's precessional frequency is 42.57 MHz/T, and it is used in clinical MRI. A few examples of hydrogen nuclei precessional frequencies at various magnetic field strengths are given below:

- 21.285 MHz at 0.5 T
- 42.57 MHz at 1 T
- 63.86 MHz at 1.5 T
- 127.71 MHz at 3 T
- 297.99 MHz at 7 T

In the electromagnetic spectrum, the range of frequencies of radio waves corresponds to the precessional frequency of hydrogen nuclei. When hydrogen nuclei are at rest or in equilibrium, their magnetic moments are out of phase with one another. In Fig. 1.7, the position of each magnetic moment of hydrogen along the circular precessional path represents this phase. In phase means that all of the individual magnetic moments of hydrogen nuclei are located along the circular precessional path in the same location.

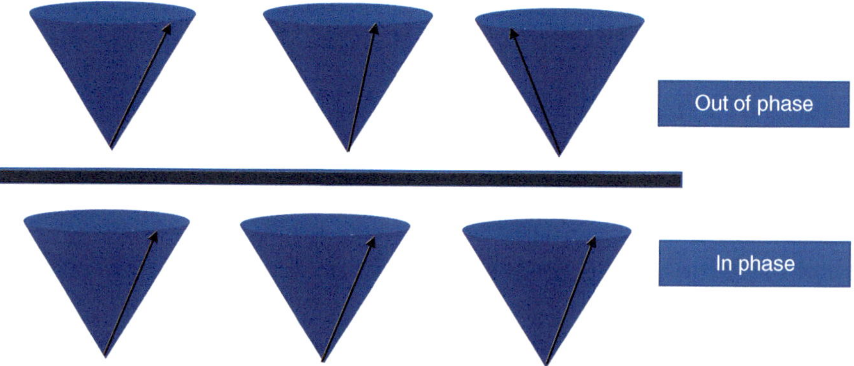

Fig. 1.7 Phase of magnetic moments of hydrogen nuclei

1.5 Resonance, Signal Generation and Image Decoding

Resonance is a process involving energy transition when an object is exposed to a frequency to its natural frequency. This resonance is induced in clinical MRI by applying a radiofrequency (RF) pulse to the main magnetic field at the exact frequency of the precessing hydrogen nuclei at 90°. This process eventually causes the hydrogen nuclei to resonate at their precessional frequency given by the Larmor equation as discussed earlier in this chapter. Because their precessional frequency and gyromagnetic ratio differ from hydrogen, other MR active nuclei do not resonate. Resonance produces two effects: energy absorption and phase coherence.

Energy absorption

The RF pulse or the excitation pulse gives enough energy to the hydrogen nuclei as depicted in Fig. 1.8. This absorption of energy at 90° to the main magnetic field causes an increase in the number of high energy or spin-up hydrogen nuclei. At a certain point, the number of spin-up nuclei equals the number of spin-down nuclei and attains a position known as the transverse plane. The transverse plane's net magnetization (NMV) is located between the two energy states. The movement of the NMV through 90° away from the main magnetic field is referred to as a flip angle, as shown in Fig. 1.9.

Phase Coherence

The absorption of energy aids the nuclei's magnetic moments in moving into phase with one another. The NMW in the transverse plane precesses at the Larmor frequency due to phase coherence and matching of both spin-up and spin-down nuclei.

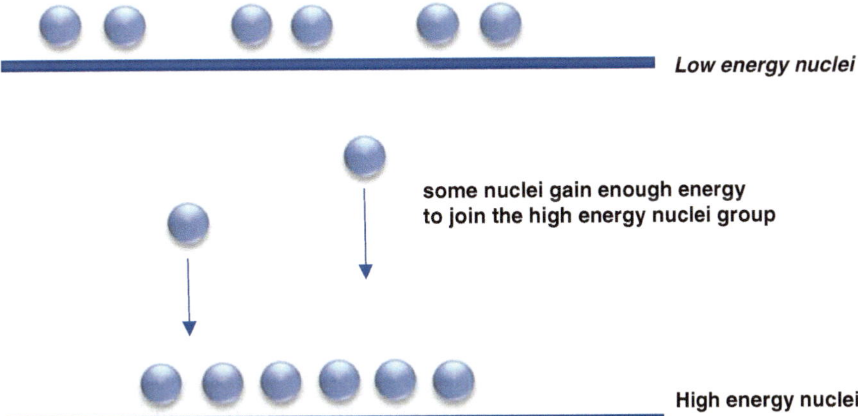

Fig. 1.8 Energy transfer process during excitation

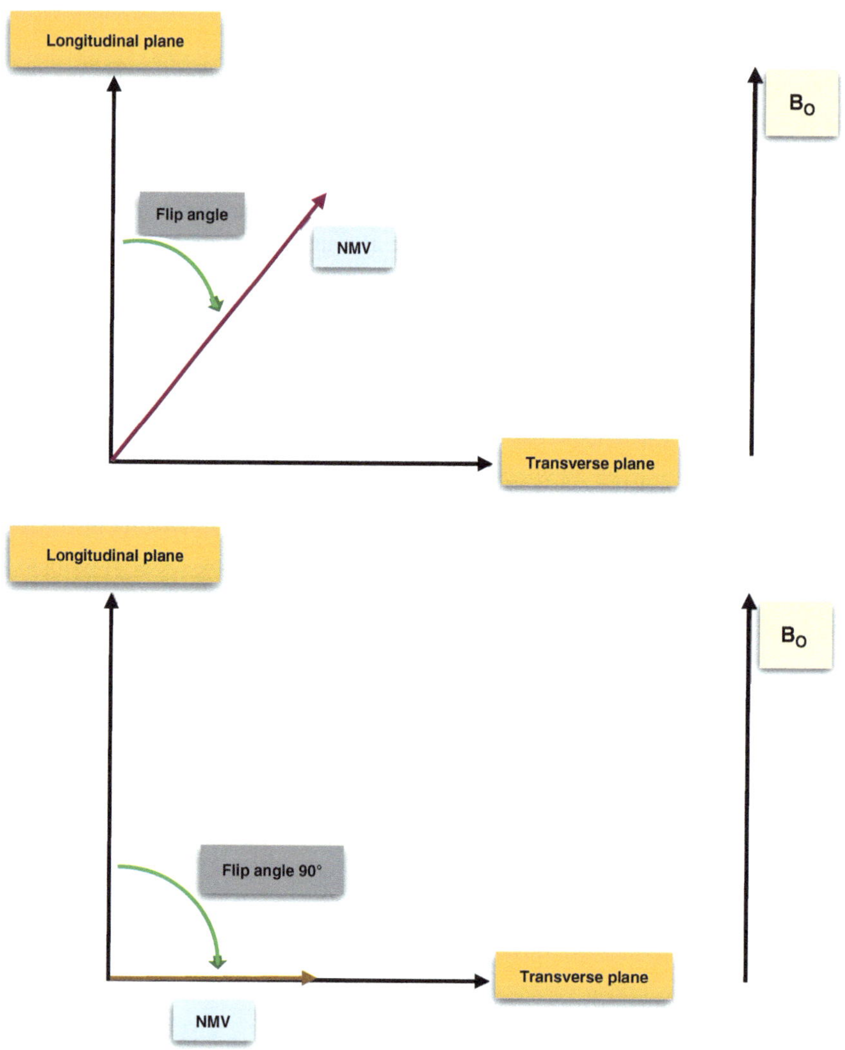

Fig. 1.9 Role of flip angle on transverse magnetization

1.5.1 The MR Signal

The magnetic moments of hydrogen nuclei precessing in the transverse plane are the result of phase coherence and energy absorption. As a result of the resonance phenomenon, the receiver coil can now be placed in the transverse plane while the NMW rotates around it, inducing a voltage in it. The MR signal is the measured voltage. The signal generated in the receiver coil begins to decrease immediately after the RF pulse is removed. In the transverse plane, the phase component of the NMV begins to decrease, as does the signal or voltage induced in the receiver coil. This is referred to as the free induction decay (FID) [20].

1.5.2 Steps in MR Image Encoding

The basics of MR encoding and signal generation can be very well understood by understanding the function of gradient coils. Gradient coils consist of wire through which electric currents are passed, to cause changes in the main magnetic field. They can cause an increase or decrease in the strength of the magnetic field linearly as depicted in Fig. 1.10. The gradient coils consist of *X*, *Y* and *Z* gradients, and they alter the magnetic field accordingly in their respective axes. These three gradients collectively perform the task of spatial encoding of the MR signal, namely, the slice selection, phase encoding and the frequency encoding [22, 23].

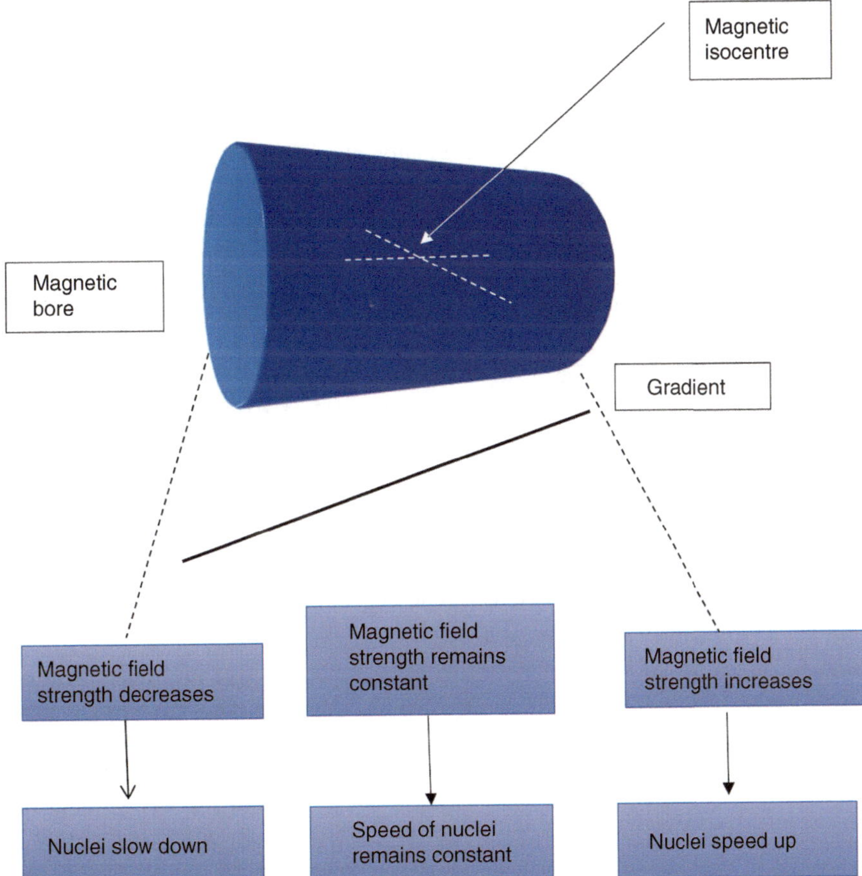

Fig. 1.10 Gradient coil system

1.6 Understanding the Physics Behind Magnetic Resonance Imaging (MRI)

The nuclear magnetic resonance principle (NMR) is based on the nucleus net magnetic moment associated with the nuclear spin. Classical physics uses NMR where it is feasible to orientate the bar magnet in the magnetic field with smooth transitions between energy states. A transition between the energy nucleus can be caused by applying an electromagnetic field (radiofrequency waves) at the resonance frequency (Larmor frequency for 1H is 42.6 MHz/T). After pulsed irradiation, this precession of transverse magnetization creates a tiny electrical signal in a coil that is then amplified and sent to the digital converter analogue. Later spatial encoding is carried out by gradients of the magnetic field resulting in distinct frequencies of resonance in space. In 2D imaging, during the implementation of a gradient in *Z*-direction ("slice selection"), the spin excitation of an image slice is conducted by irradiation with an electromagnetic field at the resonance of the slice. The second dimension is encoded with a gradient applied during signal readings in *X*-direction ("frequency selection or encoding"). Finally, the spins display distinct stages depending on their spatial location ("phase encoding") by various repetitions of the excitation readout sequence with the implementation of gradients of variable intensity in *Y*-direction. From the frequency and phase distribution ("k-space") in the MRI signal, the fast Fourier transformation can calculate the images in the position space. Water molecules from the largest composition within the human body consist of two hydrogen and one oxygen nucleus or proton. Hence, hydrogen is chosen as an MR active nucleus as it has a single solitary proton and is very abundant within the human body. The field strength of the order of 0.5–3 T is used in the superconducting variant for clinical use. The recent MR magnets provide excellent images which are of greater diagnostic value because it provides very high soft-tissue resolution. This high contrast resolution is extremely beneficial in brain imaging. However, MRI has limitations in that it provides the user with gross macroscopic details, but these abnormalities are only visible at the anatomical scale. Due to the limitations of MRI, diffusion-weighted imaging (DWI) and diffusion-tensor imaging (DTI) have gained popularity (Fig. 1.11).

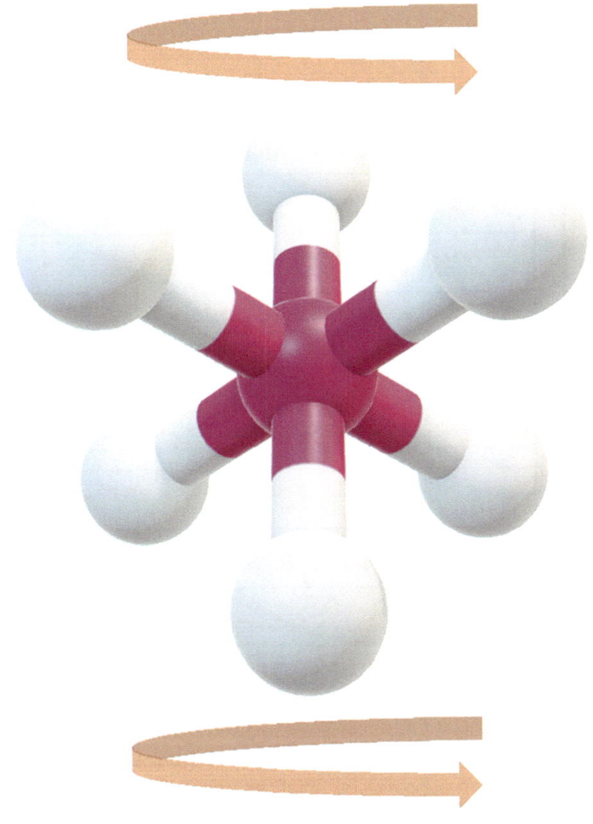

Fig. 1.11 Spin-up and spin-down nuclei

1.7 k-Space

A spin-echo formation in MRI is a result of excitation and refocusing radiofrequency (RF) pulses applied, while a gradient echo is formed due to gradient reversal on the frequency encoding axis. The echoes thus produced are known as MRI signals. The utilization in differences in relaxation times between tissues to obtain different contrast in MR images by changing imaging parameters like echo time (TE), repetition time (TR) and flip angle was demonstrated by Sir Peter Mansfield [24]. Magnetic field gradients cause a change in the magnetic field in a particular direction which helps in location encoding of the signal and hence help in slice selection, phase encoding and frequency encoding of the image [25]. k-space-filling refers to the echo signal collected row by row. However, faster filling techniques fill many lines of k-space per TR. TR refers to the time between the excitation of two RF pulses. The final image is thus formed using a 2D or 3D inverse Fourier transformation. As an overview, the centre lines of k-space contain low-frequency information, while the periphery contains high spatial frequency information [26]. The k-space-filling pattern is depicted in Fig. 1.12.

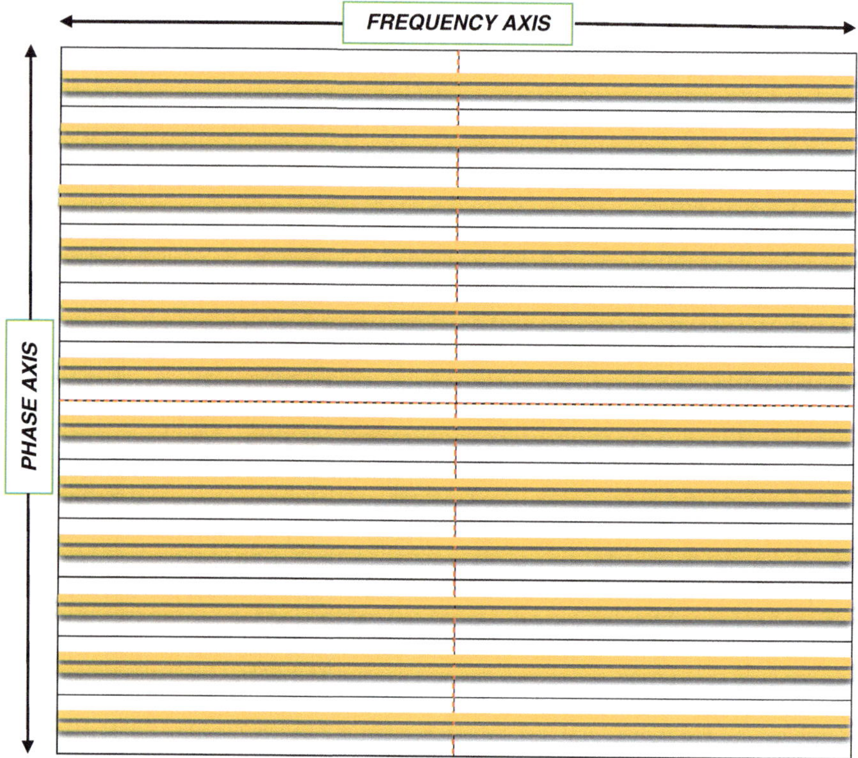

Fig. 1.12 Showing k-space-filling pattern for one slice

1.7.1 Fast Fourier Transform (FFT)

The physics and mathematics involved in fast Fourier transform form the basis of image processing in MRI. An MRI image formed depends upon the phase and frequency matrix which in turn depend upon the pixels and number of k-space lines filled. Each pixel is given a specific greyscale value depending upon its frequency and spatial location on that pixel. The FFT then converts the frequency amplitude into the frequency domain during readout.

1.7.2 k-Space Functions and Characteristics

k-Space is a rectangular, imaginary space with two axes perpendicular to each other. The horizontal axis is called frequency while the vertical one is known as the phase. k-Space is considered a spatial frequency domain because it tells us about the information from where the frequency of a signal arises from the patient, and it stores it. On the other hand, the phase axis tells us the exact position or orientation. Therefore, the unit of k-space is radians per cm.

1.7.3 Data Sampling Techniques

The three ways in which data is acquired in MRI are sequential, two-dimensional and three-dimensional. The sequential acquisition will acquire the entire data from slice one and then move to the corresponding slices. Two-dimensional acquisition acquires information to complete one line of k-space in one slice and then in successive rows to fill the same sort of information and proceed further. Three-dimensional data acquisition tries to fill the entire volume data and fill almost all the lines of k-space simultaneously.

1.7.4 k-Space Traversal

For frequency and phase encoding, k-space traversal filling is based on the polarity and amplitude of the gradients. The FOV is determined by the amplitude of the frequency encoding gradient, while the phase matrix of the image is determined by the phase encoding gradient. The polarity of the gradient describes the direction of the k-space. The positive frequency encoding gradient in k-space moves from left to right, while the positive encoding gradient fills the top half of k-space and vice versa.

1.7.5 k-Space in Pulse Sequences

The k-space-filling across the pulse sequences uses either of the techniques as mentioned below:

- Partial averaging
- Partial echo
- Rectangular FOV
- Anti-aliasing
- Fast spin echo
- Keyhole imaging
- Respiratory compensation
- Parallel imaging

k-Space Facts

- k-Space is not the final image.
- k-Space stores data in symmetrical format.
- The signal and contrast in the image is the result of central lines of k-space, while the outer lines contribute to resolution.
- Central line information contributes to signal and contrast, while exterior line information contributes to resolution.

1.8 Classification of MRI Pulse Sequences

MRI pulse sequences are mainly classified into two major groups: spin-echo and gradient-echo pulse sequences.

Spin echo is again sub-classified into the following subtypes:

1. Single and dual-spin echo
2. Fast spin echo
3. Inversion recover

Gradient-echo pulse sequences are further sub-classified in the following subtypes:

1. Steady state and weighting in gradient-echo pulse sequences
2. Coherent echo
3. Incoherent echo
4. Balanced gradient echo
5. Steady-state free precession
6. Fast gradient echo
7. Echo-planar imaging
8. Diffusion-weighted imaging [27, 28]
9. Diffusion tensor EPI sequences (spin or gradient echo based)

1.9 Basic Pulse Timing Parameters

Figure 1.13 depicts a pulse sequence as a planned timing combination of RF pulses, signal generation and RF recovery times. The time of repetition (TR) and time of echo (TE) are critical components of a pulse sequence (TE). TR denotes the time interval between the application of one RF pulse and the application of the next RF pulse. TR is in charge of the amount of T1 weighting. However, as explained earlier in this chapter, TE is the time interval between the application of one RF pulse and the peak of the signal induced in the receiver coil. The amount of T2 weighting is controlled by TE, which will be discussed in Chap. 2.

Summary: In this chapter, we have introduced the history and basic principles of magnetic resonance imaging. In Chap. 2, we shall be discussing the image contrast mechanisms in diffusion-weighted and diffusion-tensor imaging in detail.

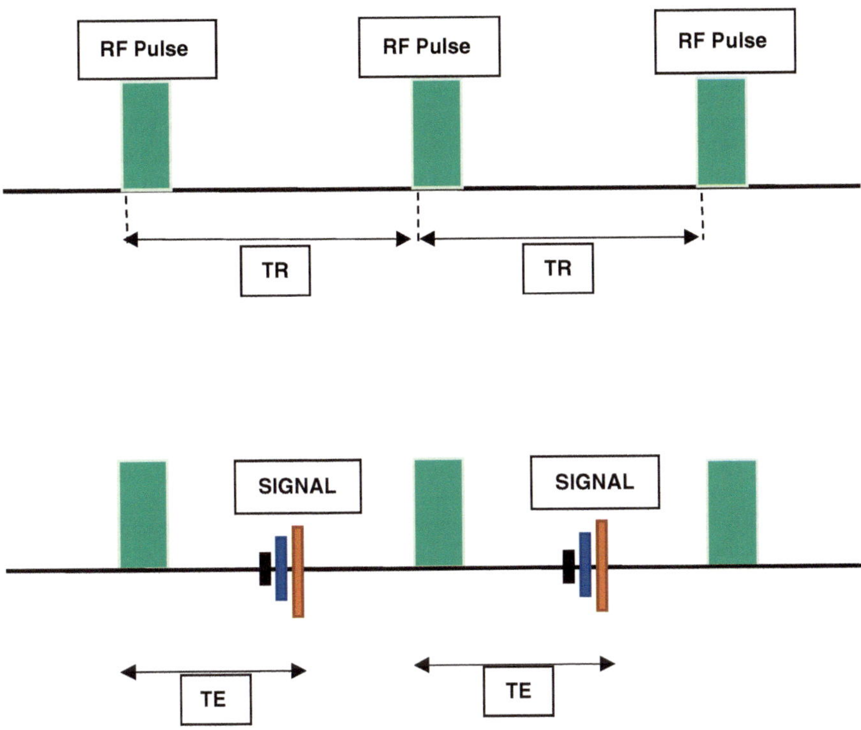

Fig. 1.13 Basic pulse timing sequence and pattern

References

1. White N. Quantitative diffusion magnetic resonance imaging of the brain: validation, acquisition, and analysis. UC San Diego. 2010. ProQuest ID: White_ucsd_0033D_10706. Merritt ID: ark:/20775/bb60763753. Retrieved from https://escholarship.org/uc/item/5ss7j07v.
2. Brown R, Bennett JJ. The miscellaneous botanical works of Robert Brown ... The miscellaneous botanical works of Robert Brown ... Published for the Ray society by R. Hardwicke. 2012. https://doi.org/10.5962/bhl.title.55658.
3. Carr H, Purcell E. Effects of diffusion on free precession in nuclear magnetic resonance experiments. Phys Rev. 1954;94(3):630–8. http://link.aps.org/doi/10.1103/PhysRev.94.630.
4. Hrabe J, Kaur G, Guilfoyle DN. Principles and limitations of NMR diffusion measurements. J Med Phys. 2007;32(1):34–42. https://pubmed.ncbi.nlm.nih.gov/21217917.
5. Clark CA, Le Bihan D. Water diffusion compartmentation and anisotropy at high b values in the human brain. Magn Reson Med. 2000;44(6):852–9. http://www.ncbi.nlm.nih.gov/pubmed/11108621.
6. Lauterbur PC. Image formation by induced local interactions. Examples employing nuclear magnetic resonance. 1973. Clin Orthop Relat Res. 1989;244:3–6. http://www.ncbi.nlm.nih.gov/pubmed/2663289.
7. Damadian R, Goldsmith M, Minkoff L. NMR in cancer: XVI. FONAR image of the live human body. Physiol Chem Phys. 1977;9(1):97–100, 108. http://www.ncbi.nlm.nih.gov/pubmed/909957.

8. Hunsche S, Moseley ME, Stoeter P, Hedehus M. Diffusion-tensor MR imaging at 1.5 and 3.0 T: initial observations. Radiology. 2001;221(2):550–6. http://pubs.rsna.org/doi/abs/10.1148/radiol.2212001823.
9. Hunsche S, Moseley ME, Stoeter P, Hedehus M. Diffusion-tensor MR imaging at 1.5 and 3.0 T: initial observations. Radiology. 2001;221(2):550–6. http://www.ncbi.nlm.nih.gov/pubmed/11687703.
10. Edelman RR. The history of MR imaging as seen through the pages of radiology. Radiology. 2014;273(2):181–200.
11. Stehling MK, Schmitt F, Ladebeck R. Echo-planar MR imaging of human brain oxygenation changes. J Magn Reson Imaging. 1993;3(3):471–4.
12. Edelman RR, Wielopolski P, Schmitt F. Echo-planar MR imaging. Radiology. 1994;192(3):600–12.
13. Deshmane A, Gulani V, Griswold MA. HHS Public Access. 2015;36(1):55–72.
14. Yamanaka K. MRI parallel imaging. Jpn J Clin Radiol. 2002;47(13):1779–88.
15. Hamilton J, Franson D, Seiberlich N. Recent advances in parallel imaging for MRI. Prog Nucl Magn Reson Spectrosc. 2017;101:71–95.
16. Whinder F. One man and his machine. Lancet Neurol. 2013;12(6):537.
17. Faro SH, Haughton V, Mohamed FB. Functional MRI: basic principles and clinical applications. New York: Springer; 2006.
18. Glover GH. MRI: basic principles and future potential. Comput Aided Surg. 2000;5(2):132.
19. Dale BM, Brown MA, Semelka RC. MRI: basic principles and applications. John Wiley & Sons; 2015.
20. Sharma HA. MRI physics–basic principles. Acta Neuropsychiatrica. 2009;21(4):200–1.
21. Nayak SM. MRI: basic principles and applications. Radiology. 1996;200:1.
22. Tyler P, Butt S. Basic principles of MRI. In: Radionuclide and hybrid bone imaging. Berlin: Springer; 2012. p. 149–71.
23. Tang C, Brown MA, Semelka RC. MRI: Basic Principles and Applications. Radiat Res. 1996;145(2):243.
24. Mansfield P. Multi-planar image formation using NMR spin echoes. J Phys C Solid State Phys. 1977;10(3):L55–8. http://stacks.iop.org/0022-3719/10/i=3/a=004?key=crossref.f48893f3d8bf21cb4a102c6293b5ce83.
25. Lauterbur PC. The Classic: Image Formation by Induced Local Interactions: Examples Employing Nuclear Magnetic Resonance. Clinical Orthopaedics and Related Research®. 1989;244:3–6.
26. Stoffey RD, Mizrachi JS. In: Catherine W, Carolyn KR, Talbot J, editors. MRI in practice, 4th ed. West Sussex, UK: Wiley-Blackwell, 456 pp., 2011. $51.99 softcover (ISBN: 978-1444337433). Am J Roentgenol. 2012;198(5).
27. Fong W. Handbook of MRI pulse sequences. Med Phys. 2005;32(5):1452.
28. Bernstein MA, King KF, Zhou XJ. Handbook of MRI pulse sequences. Amsterdam: Elsevier; 2004.

2 Image Contrast Mechanisms in Diffusion-Weighted and Diffusion-Tensor Imaging

The previous chapter discussed the fundamentals of magnetic resonance imaging as well as its applications in brain grey- and white-matter imaging. The major learning point was the use of a single solitary hydrogen proton for MR imaging. The concepts of MR active nucleus and its utilization to form an image of the human body with the help of magnets, gradient coils, radiofrequency coils and image encoding were also discussed. In the current chapter, we will study the various components of image contrast and weighting employed in magnetic resonance imaging in detail. Image weighting and contrast play a vital role in interpreting MR images, unlike other counterpart imaging modalities which possess standard image contrast. MRI varies in image weighting and contrast for individual pulse sequences which in turn depend upon key parameters like time of repetition (TR), time of echo (TE), turbo factor, time of inversion (TI), the *b*-value and flip angle which are also known as extrinsic contrast parameters. The intrinsic contrast parameters affecting MRI image contrast are the apparent diffusion coefficient (ADC), T1 recovery, T2 decay, proton density (PD) and flow. Hence, understanding this mechanism forms the basis for interpreting clinical images in MRI.

2.1 What Do We Understand by Image Contrast in MRI?

The excellent soft-tissue contrast resolution exhibited by MRI makes it the modality of choice for imaging compared to its counterparts which utilize ionizing radiation for image acquisition. However, contrast mechanisms in MRI are complex because many variables contribute to image contrast. Hence, a deep understanding of these factors becomes instrumental in learning contrast mechanisms in routine MRI and advanced techniques like diffusion-weighted and diffusion-tensor imaging.

Every image generated in MRI has contrast and is divided into two types: high signal and low signal images. High signal depicts areas of white on the image,

R. P. Kotian, P. Koteshwar, *Diffusion Tensor Imaging and Fractional Anisotropy*,
https://doi.org/10.1007/978-981-19-5001-8_2

whereas low signal depicts areas of black (dark) on the image. The in-between image depicts various shades of grey that fall between white and black images. We can now equate this with the body tissue and transverse component of the net magnetization vector (NMV). A tissue depicts a higher signal on the image if it possesses a larger component of the transverse magnetization, and a lower signal is a result of a small component of transverse magnetization. The contrast component of MRI is well explained by the two extremes in the human body, namely, fat and water.

2.1.1 MRI-Specific Composition and Characteristics of Fat and Water in the Human Body

Why choose only fat and water for MR image contrast? Clinical MRI extracts signal from hydrogen protons as discussed in Chap. 1, and the sole reason is its large abundance which comprises 90% of nuclei in the human body. This single solitary hydrogen proton thus detected can either be a part of water molecules such as fats, proteins or carbohydrates. By further exploiting these characteristics of hydrogen nuclei, MRI gives excellent soft-tissue contrast resolution irrespective of its bonding with water or fat. Let us now discuss the composition of fat and water in the human body. Fat mainly consists of hydrogen atoms attached to carbon comprising very large molecules. This larger structure results in a slow rate of molecular motion. To conclude, fat has lower inherent energy making it possible to absorb energy very efficiently. Water on the other hand consists of smaller molecules linked to oxygen comprising of a higher rate of molecular motion. This property leads to higher inherent energy and reduced absorption of energy. The above-mentioned differences in fat and water produce different image contrast in body tissues due to their relaxation times [1]. Figure 2.1 depicts the magnitude of transverse magnetization on the signal generated in fat and water, respectively.

A basic pulse sequence consists of a predetermined flip angle with an RF pulse, which causes transverse magnetization and signal generation in the receiver coil. However, once the RF excitation pulse is removed, the signal in the receiver coil begins to decrease as the NMV begins to realign back to the longitudinal magnetization from the transverse plane. This results in a decrease in the signal voltage detected by the receiver coil. This is known as free induction decay (FID). The NMV in the transverse plane decreases as a result of field inhomogeneities and relaxation processes that vary by tissue. The understanding of FID becomes very crucial when we discuss complex imaging techniques in the coming chapters of diffusion-weighted and diffusion-tensor imaging. The concept of T1 recovery and T2 decay will be shortly discussed in the upcoming subsection. However, the concept of T2* (T2* star) will be introduced at this moment. Even though inhomogeneities in the external magnetic field cause alterations to it, every attempt in MR imaging focuses primarily on the uniformity of the main magnetic field. The removal of the RF excitation pulse causes transverse magnetization decay, and this exponential decay process is known as T2*. T2* is a combination of T2 decay itself and the magnetic field inhomogeneities around its surrounding [2].

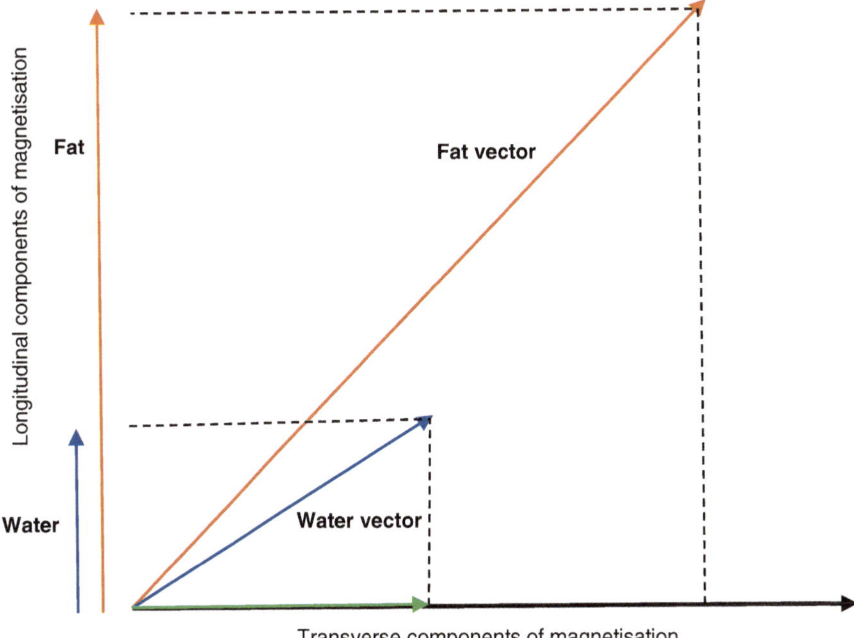

Fig. 2.1 Component of transverse magnetization in fat and water

2.1.2 What Is T1 Recovery? Process of T1 Recovery in Fat and Water

The net effect of the RF pulse withdrawal has several effects. To begin, the nuclei emit energy from the RF pulse via a process known as spin-lattice energy transfer. The NMV then recovers and aligns itself to the main magnetic field. This exchange of energy between the nuclei and its surrounding environment or lattice is called T1 recovery. The entire process of T1 recovery differs in different tissue types. Every tissue will possess its own T1 time, and it is an inherent tissue-specific property. T1 time, also known as T1 recovery, is the amount of time it takes for 63% of the longitudinal magnetization to recover after the RF excitation pulse is removed. TR is defined as the time elapsed between the application of one RF pulse and the next, and TR determines the TI recovery of any given tissue.

2.1.2.1 T1 Recovery in Fat (T1 Relaxation)

T1 relaxation is the process by which nuclei begin exchanging the energy provided by the RF to the surrounding environment. Fat is comprised of larger molecules as discussed earlier. Hence, the fat nuclei quickly dispose of the energy to the surrounding given by the RF pulse and return to B_0 quickly. Therefore, the T1 time or T1 recovery of fat is very short as depicted in Fig. 2.2.

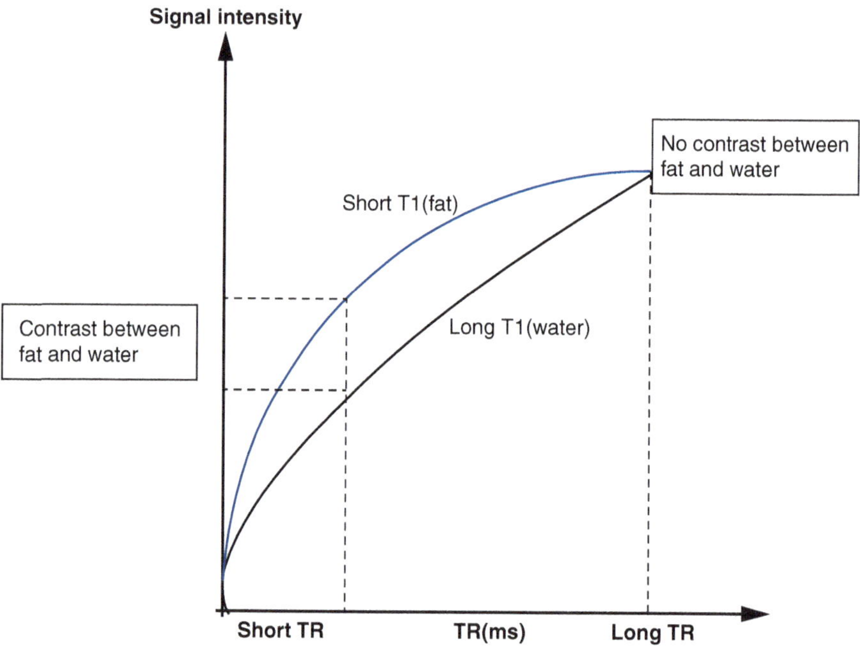

Fig. 2.2 T1 differences between fat and water

2.1.2.2 T1 Recovery in Water (T1 Relaxation)

Water is comprised of smaller molecules and is inefficient at absorbing or receiving energy. Hence, water nuclei do not quickly dispose of their energy to the surrounding given by the RF pulse and do not return to B_0 quickly. Therefore, the T1 time or T1 recovery of water is long as depicted in Fig. 2.2. The TR regulates the NMV in both fat and water after it has recovered before the next RF is applied. The use of short TRs does not allow full longitudinal recovery in both fat and water resulting in different longitudinal components in both water and fat. This results in different individual transverse components in fat and water after the application of the next RF pulse. Because of differences in T1 recovery, this process is known as saturation, and it results in a contrast difference between fat and water. Because long TRs allow for full recovery of the longitudinal components in fat and water, no contrast difference between fat and water is observed. It is very important to understand that T1 recovery and T2 decay are two processes that are independent of each other and will be explained in the next subsection [3].

2.1.3 What Is T2 Decay? Process of T2 Decay in Fat and Water

T2 decay occurs when the in-phase transverse magnetization begins to dephase after the RF excitation pulse is removed. T2 decay is the name given to this process. The hydrogen nuclei lose phase coherence due to energy exchange with adjacent nuclei (spin-spin energy transfer mechanism) and inhomogeneities in the external magnetic field. This is an exponential process that occurs at different times in different tissues. The T2 decay time in tissue is an intrinsic contrast parameter that is defined as the time it takes for 63% of the transverse magnetization to be lost due to the dephasing process [3].

2.1.3.1 T2 Decay in Fat (T2 Decay)

The energy exchange between neighbouring nuclei is very efficient in fat molecules, and it also possesses a compact packing structure. As this energy exchange process is quick in fat, it has a short T2 time compared to water as shown in Fig. 2.3.

2.1.3.2 T2 Decay in Water (T2 Decay)

The energy exchange time in the water is comparatively less efficient as compared to fat. Hence, the T2 time of water is long as depicted in Fig. 2.3. The time of excitation (TE) is defined as the time elapsed between the application of one RF pulse and the peak of the signal induced in the receiver coil. TE is also responsible for the amount of transverse magnetization for decay manifestation in fat and water. Hence, the TE controls the amount of T2 decay in a particular tissue. Figure 2.3 demarcates the significance of using a long TE to visualize larger contrast differences in fat and water using long TEs. The use of short TEs prevents full dephasing in fat or water,

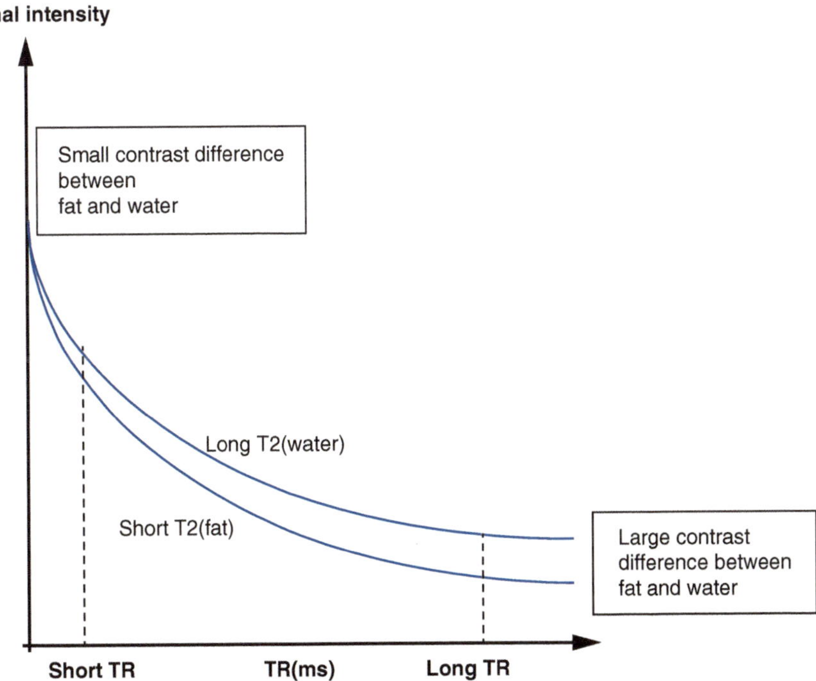

Fig. 2.3 T2 differences between fat and water

resulting in transverse components that are similar. Hence, using short TEs results in very small contrast differences between fat and water. To conclude, fat and water are the two extremes for MR imaging in image contrast. All other tissues within the human body exhibit different contrast mechanisms which fall in between fat and water contrast, respectively [4].

2.1.4 What Is T1 Weighting? How Are T1-Weighted Images Formed?

The intrinsic contrast mechanisms of the tissue (T1, T2 and proton density) affect image contrast in MRI regardless of the pulse sequence used or its extrinsic contrast parameters such as the TR and TE. The two extremes in MRI are fat and water, where they might appear bright or dark depending on the pulse sequence and the selected extrinsic contrast parameters. Thus, image weighting is defined as the process of predicting the image contrast of a specific tissue by selecting or weighting the image towards one contrast mechanism (T1) and away from the other two, namely, T2 and proton density PD.

T1 relaxation time differences between tissues should be visible on a T1-weighted image. To achieve T1 weighting, a short TR is used to ensure that the NMW in fat and water do not relax and realign back to the position of the external magnetic field before the next RF pulse is applied. The application of a longer TR will cause both the fat and water to gain full T1 recovery, and no contrast differences will be noticeable between them. The contrast of a T1-weighted image is primarily determined by differences in tissue T1 recovery times. TR is the main governing parameter affecting T1-weighted images. To diminish the T2 effects in a T1-weighted image, the TE must be short. The TR and TE of a T1-weighted image are both short. Tissues with short T1 relaxation times, like fat, appear bright on the T1-weighted MR image, whereas water has long T1 relaxation times and appears dark. T1-weighted images depict anatomy but also can demonstrate pathology when used with a gadolinium-based contrast agent [1, 3] (Fig. 2.4).

2.1.5 What Is T2 Weighting? How Are T2-Weighted Images Formed?

The intrinsic contrast mechanisms of the tissue (T1, T2 and proton density) affect image contrast in MRI regardless of the pulse sequence used or its extrinsic contrast parameters such as the TR and TE. The two extremes in MRI are fat and water, where they might appear bright or dark depending on the pulse sequence and the selected extrinsic contrast parameters. Thus, image weighting is defined as the process of predicting the image contrast of a specific tissue by selecting or weighting the image towards one contrast mechanism (T2) and away from the other two, namely, T1 and proton density PD.

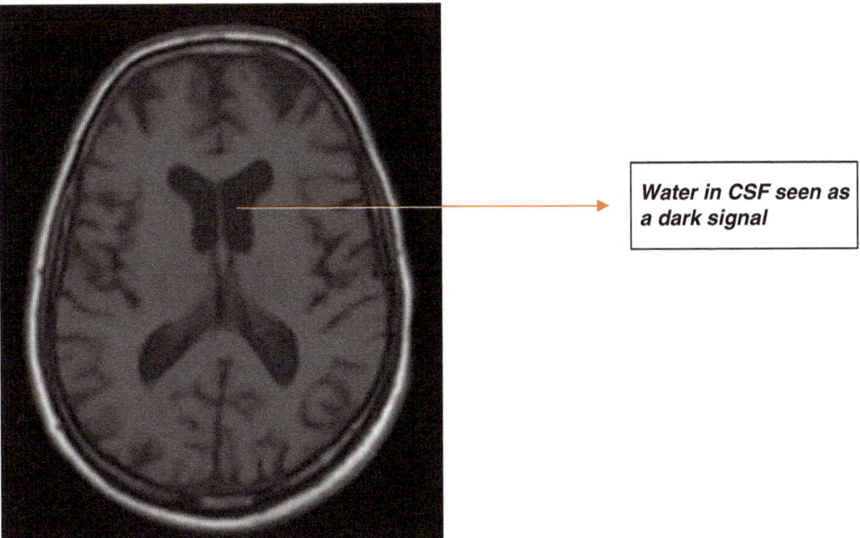

Fig. 2.4 T1-weighted image

The differences in the T2 relaxation times of tissues should be visible on a T2-weighted image. A long TE is employed to achieve T2 weighting to ensure that the NMW in fat and water has had time to decay. The application of a short TE will not give time for both the fat and water to decay, and no contrast differences in their T2 times will be noticeable between them.

The contrast of a T2-weighted image is primarily determined by differences in the tissue's T2 decay times. TE is the main governing parameter affecting T2-weighted images. To diminish the T1 effects in a T2-weighted image, the TR must be long. A long TE and long TR characterize a T2-weighted image. Figure 2.5 depicts how tissues with short T2 decay times, such as fat, appear dark on the T2-weighted MR image, whereas water with long T2 decay times appears bright. T2-weighted images depict pathology as water is the main component in various pathological conditions and appears bright on T2-weighted images [1, 3].

2.1.6 Proton Density Image Formation by Masking T1 and T2 Weighting

The intrinsic contrast mechanisms of the tissue (T1, T2 and proton density) affect image contrast in MRI regardless of the pulse sequence used or its extrinsic contrast parameters like the TR and TE. The two extremes in MRI are fat and water, where they might appear bright or dark depending on the pulse sequence and the selected extrinsic contrast parameters. Thus, image weighting is defined as the process of predicting the image contrast of a specific tissue by selecting or weighting the image

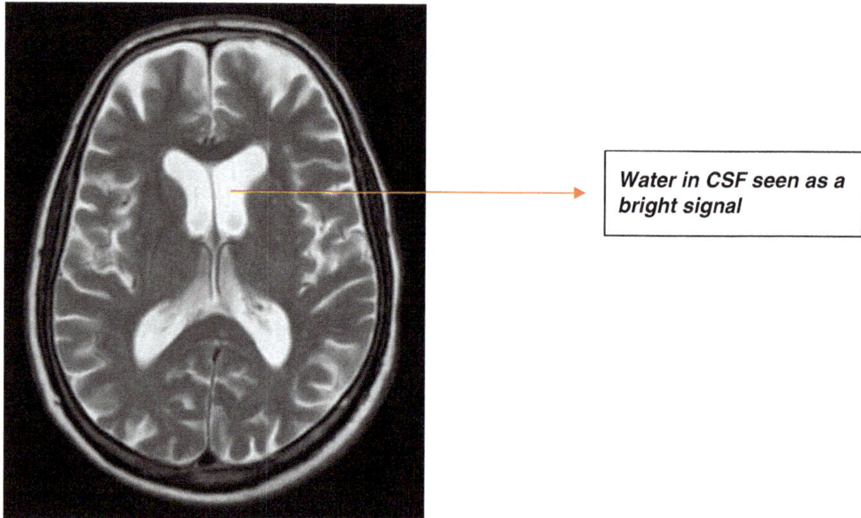

Fig. 2.5 T2-weighted image

towards one contrast mechanism (PD) and away from the other two, namely, T1 and T2.

In contrast to the T1 relaxation and T2 decay times of the tissue in T1-W and T2-W images, the PD-weighted image is determined by differences in the total number of hydrogen protons in the tissue. As a result, a proton-weighted image contrast is determined by differences in the proton density of the tissues. Tissues with a high proton density depict bright signals, while low proton density areas depict dark signals as depicted in Fig. 2.6. This process is directly related to the amount of transverse magnetization of the tissues. To obtain PD-weighted images, both the T1 and T2 effects must be reduced. T1 effects are reduced when a long TR is chosen, whereas T2 effects are reduced when a short TR is chosen. The cortical bone is an important learning point. It always appears dark with a low signal on MR images regardless of weighting because it is composed of low proton density. PD-weighted images show anatomy and pathology in certain areas of the human body. In recent times, PD imaging is mainly done to visualize the cartilages, ligaments and tendons, respectively [3].

Fig. 2.6 PD-weighted image

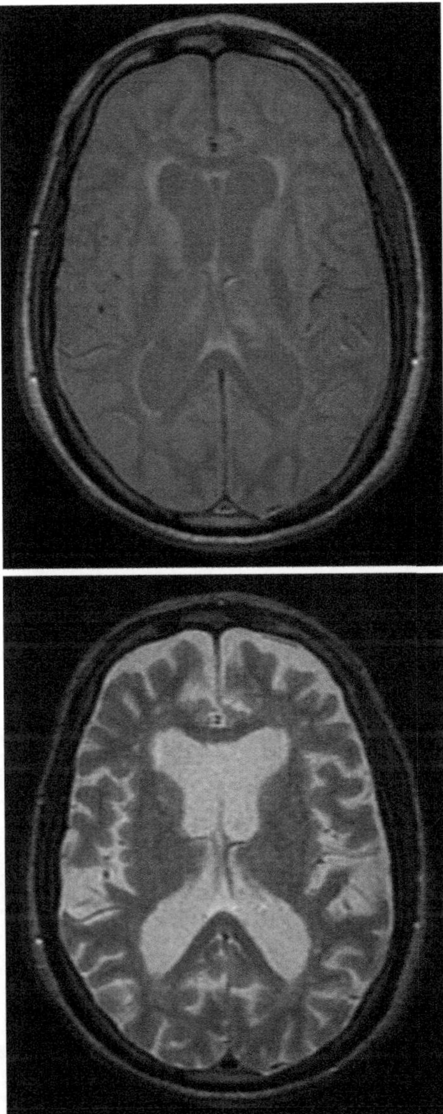

2.2 Mechanisms of Image Contrast in Diffusion-Weighted Imaging (DWI)

Tissue permeability is very well demonstrated by its ability to diffuse through cell structure. This is calculated using the apparent diffusion coefficient (ADC) in DWI. This parameter is not influenced by other extrinsic and intrinsic parameters that affect conventional MR imaging, and all these calculations are done using computer software. The speciality of ADC is that it appears exactly the reverse of DWI [5].

Diffusion gradients can be used to create DW images, but the signal intensity and image contrast are affected by the apparent diffusion coefficient (ADC). Because liquids have a high ADC, they appear bright or hyperintense. At least two diffusion-weighted measurements with different *b*-values are required to calculate ADC. As a result, the ADC can be calculated accurately by determining the signal intensity at the higher and lower *b*-values. The mean signal intensities in the region of interest for each pixel are used to create an ADC map [6].

"Image contrast in DWI can be confusing with a mix of different contrasts on display. Most of the DWI pulse sequences employ long echo times between 50 and 125 ms due to the prolonged diffusion process. Thus, diffusion-weighted images are referred to as T2 weighted, and it sometimes becomes difficult to differentiate between diffusion and T2 effects as depicted in Fig. 2.7. This causes misrepresentation of normal anatomy and pathology in the brain MRI known as T2 shine-through effect" [7, 8]. Another major disadvantage of using long echo times is the low signal-to-noise ratio of DW images. Hence diffusion weighting reduces the signal from tissues that are not liquids which result in low signal intensity on DWI. Hence, most of the newer MRI pulse sequences employ signal intensity increasing techniques. ADC calculation can also be corrected by decreasing the signal-to-noise ratio at a *b*-value higher than 1000 [9, 10]. The learning point of image contrast in DWI implies that diffusion deficit areas will always remain hyperintense (bright signal) after the application of diffusion-weighted gradients.

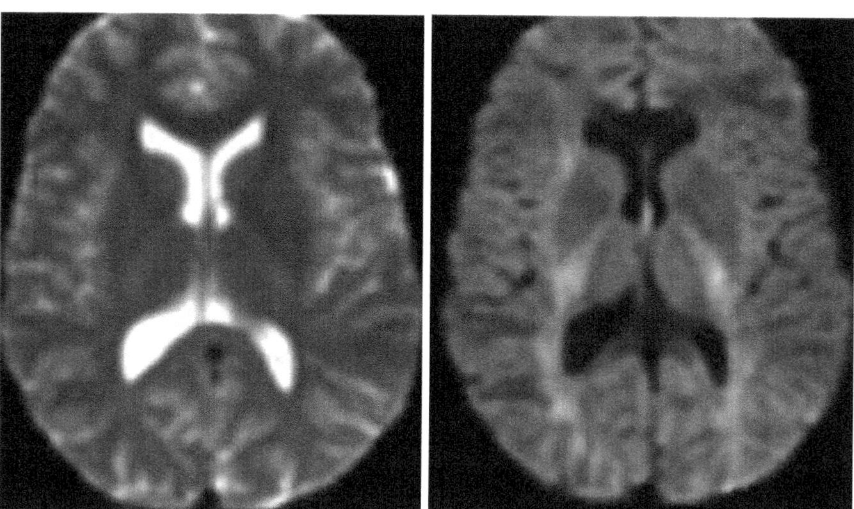

Fig. 2.7 T2-weighted and diffusion-weighted image

2.3 DTI-Based Scalar Derivative Fractional Anisotropy (FA) and Its Corresponding Image Contrast Mechanisms

The diffusion-tensor imaging (DTI)-based apparent diffusion coefficient (ADC) and fractional anisotropy (FA) maps can be visualized in the same way as conventional MRI using an 8-bit (greyscale) to 24-bit (red/green/blue colour scheme presentation) image. The region of interest (ROI) and manual drawing techniques can be employed to obtain ADC and FA values and their corresponding colour-coded maps. The concepts learned earlier in this chapter will be very instrumental in understanding the more complex image contrast mechanisms employed in diffusion-tensor imaging and FA [11].

The simplest way to understand image contrast mechanisms in DTI would be to break them into simpler components of DTI produced images. Image contrast mechanisms obtained from DTI can be mainly classified into the following: T2-weighted image or reference image, ADC or trace image, FA image and FA colour-coded maps as depicted in Fig. 2.8. The practical way of analysing image contrast and obtaining FA values for detecting pathologies within the body or specific anatomic location comprises of the following steps:

1. A T1- or T2-weighted image is obtained for anatomy visualization.
2. DTI sequence employing a fixed *b*-value and TE combination is obtained.

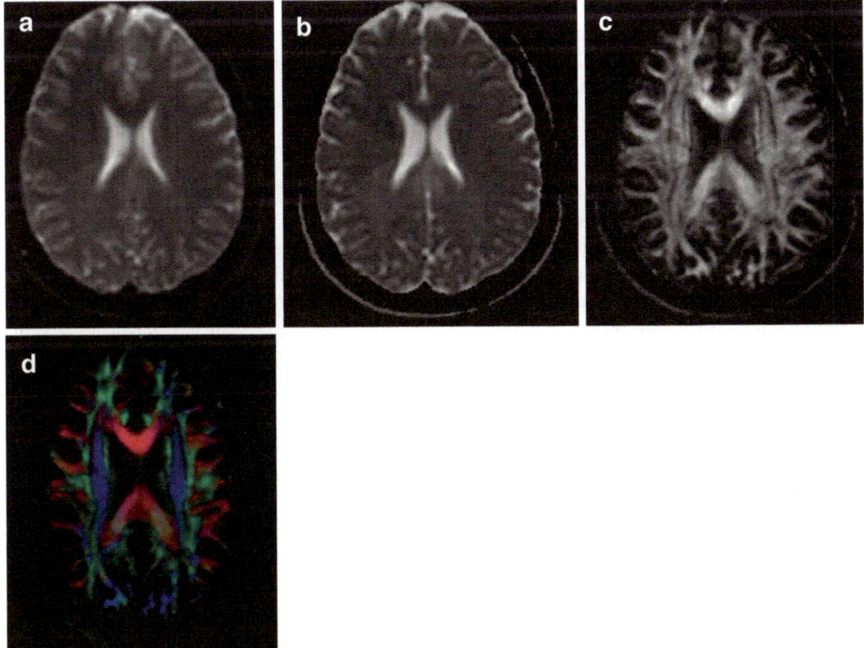

Fig. 2.8 (**a**) T2-W reference image; (**b**) trace or ADC image; (**c**) FA image; (**d**) FA colour map

3. The FA map or colour-coded FA thus obtained lack anatomical correlation.
4. DTI-derived colour-coded FA images are now overlapped with a T1- or T2-W image sequence for anatomical identification.
5. ROIs are now drawn on these overlapped images of FA+ T1-W or T2-W images to obtain FA values at the specific anatomic location, e.g. brain.
6. These FA values can be compared with a population to judge if they are high or low and predict neuro-related disorders early and aid in their treatment.

In this chapter, we discussed image contrast mechanisms in T1-, T2- and PD-weighted images, as well as DWI and DTI. In Chap. 3, we will discuss the physics of diffusion-weighted imaging in-depth.

References

1. Bley TA, Wieben O, François CJ, Brittain JH, Reeder SB. Fat and water magnetic resonance imaging. J Magn Reson Imaging. 2010;31(1):4–18.
2. Westbrook C, Roth CK, Talbot J. MRI in practice. 4th ed. New York: Wiley; 2011.
3. Foreman K. In: Westbrook C, editors. MRI at a glance, 2nd ed. Malden, MA: Wiley-Blackwell, 136 pp., 2010. $42.99 softcover (ISBN: 978-1405192552). Am J Roentgenol. 2011;196(6).
4. Stoffey RD, Mizrachi JS. In: Westbrook C, Roth CK, Talbot J, editors. MRI in practice, 4th ed. West Sussex, UK: Wiley-Blackwell, 456 pp., 2011. $51.99 softcover (ISBN: 978-1444337433). Am J Roentgenol. 2012;198(5).
5. Neil JJ. Diffusion imaging concepts for clinicians. J Magn Reson Imaging. 2008;27(1):1–7. http://www.ncbi.nlm.nih.gov/pubmed/18050325.
6. Nitz WR, Reimer P. Contrast mechanisms in MR imaging. Eur Radiol. 1999;9(6):1032–46.
7. Burdette JH, Durden DD, Elster AD, Yen YF. High b-value diffusion-weighted MRI of normal brain. J Comput Assist Tomogr. 2001;25(4):515–9. http://www.ncbi.nlm.nih.gov/pubmed/11473179.
8. Chepuri NB, Yen Y, Burdette JH, Li H, Moody DM, Maldjian JA. Diffusion anisotropy in the corpus callosum. AJNR Am J Neuroradiol. 2002;23(5):803–8.
9. Lenglet C. Brain mapping. Amsterdam: Elsevier; 2015. p. 245–51. http://www.sciencedirect.com/science/article/pii/B9780123970251002918.
10. Shen J-M, Xia X-W, Kang W-G, Yuan J-J, Sheng L. The use of MRI apparent diffusion coefficient (ADC) in monitoring the development of brain infarction. BMC Med Imaging. 2011;11(1):2. http://www.pubmedcentral.nih.gov/articlerender.fcgi?artid=3022840&tool=pmcentrez&rendertype=abstract.
11. Mori S. New image contrasts from diffusion tensor imaging: theory, meaning, and usefulness of DTI-based image contrast. In: Introduction to diffusion tensor imaging. Amsterdam: Elsevier; 2007. p. 69–84.

3 DWI Physics and Imaging Techniques

This chapter deals with basic physics related to the microstructural Brownian motion of water molecules. The techniques related to diffusion-weighted imaging probe the movement of tissue microstructure which is reflected by its freedom of motion of water molecules. The apparent diffusion coefficient (ADC) maps are free from the effects of T1 and T2 relaxation. Diffusion-weighted imaging (DWI) gives us information on the restricted flow areas within the brain but does not give us accurate length and direction. However, diffusion tensor imaging (DTI) allows us to measure the length and direction of the diffusion anisotropy of water molecules in vivo. Parallel imaging and echo-planar imaging (EPI) techniques employing quick data acquisition with reduced artefacts are employed in DWI and DTI.

3.1 Physics from Diffusion-Weighted to Diffusion-Tensor Imaging

The human brain exhibits a very complex structure of white matter (WM) comprising of neuronal axons which are parallel to one another. Its main role is the transport of outgoing signals facilitating neuronal communication [1]. WM also contains macroglial and microglial cells. Macroglial cells mainly produce myelin sheath which supports WM, regulate ion concentration and maintain blood-brain barrier, while microglial cells engulf dead cells and waste products [2–4]. For healthy brain functioning, the balance between WM cells is very necessary [5]. Glial cells are considered biomarkers in various pathologies in the neurodegenerative disorders [6]. Disturbance in axonal arrangement and transport mechanism is critical in detecting neurodegenerative disorders. The structure of a normal axon is depicted in the figure. Hence the use of diffusion of water molecules in diffusion-weighted imaging (DWI) to quantify the overall movement in WM has become a gold standard in medical imaging for diagnosis (Fig. 3.1).

R. P. Kotian, P. Koteshwar, *Diffusion Tensor Imaging and Fractional Anisotropy*,
https://doi.org/10.1007/978-981-19-5001-8_3

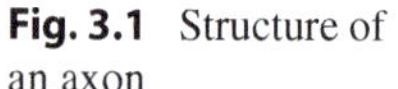
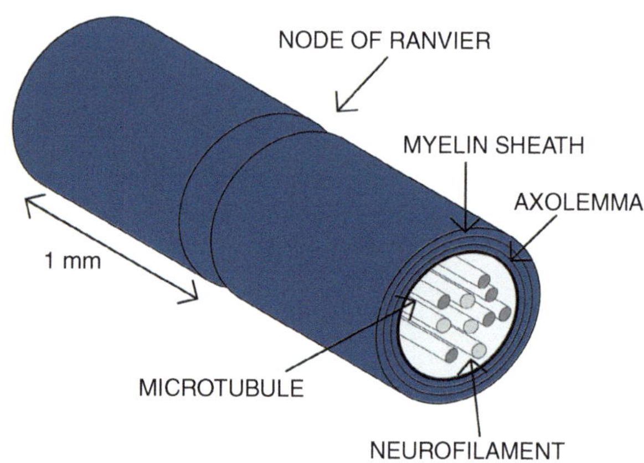

Fig. 3.1 Structure of an axon

3.2 Introduction to Diffusion-Weighted Imaging (DWI)

Diffusion-weighted imaging (DWI) is a type of magnetic resonance imaging (MR imaging) that measures Brownian motion within a tissue voxel. Diffusion, as used in diffusion-weighted imaging (DWI), refers to the random thermal motion of molecules in liquids and gases, also known as Brownian motion. The size, environment and temperature of the molecules or atoms under consideration define this motion. As a result, diffusion measurements can be used to learn about the microstructure of tissues. In the 1950 NMR experiment, Sir E.L. Hahn recognized this theory [7, 8], long before the invention of magnetic resonance imaging. In the years that followed, several significant inventions depicting quantitative measurement of the diffusion coefficient were reported [9–11]. Among these, Stejskal and Tanner's proposed theories on pulsed gradient spin echo in 1965 gained significant importance in DWI [12, 13].

The last decade has seen a tremendous improvement in DWI to visualize the random microscopic motion of water molecules. DWI techniques are used as a clinical application not only for ischemia but also in other diseases like Parkinson's disease, dyslexia, trauma or schizophrenia [14–19].

3.2.1 Physics Behind Diffusion

Earlier, DWI was not considered a useful diagnostic tool because of its artefact producing nature. Since the introduction of fast imaging sequences and techniques, DWI has been used for functional and structural imaging of biological tissues. DWI is considered as a gold standard for any neurological imaging and most importantly for the evaluation of stroke since the 1980s [20–22].

3.2.2 Brownian Motion

All molecules in liquids and gases move randomly at microscopic scales. Sir Robert Brown observed pollen grains as tiny particles within grains that moved randomly through his microscope in 1827. Brownian motion is the name given to this random molecular motion [23, 24]. Water accounts for approximately 80% of the human body. Diffusion, also known as Brownian motion, is the process of displacement of water molecules caused by collisions with surrounding compartments, and it is a thermally driven process [25]. Brownian motion is a diffusion property that reflects the random motion of molecules within a cell [26]. In a homogeneous medium, isotropic diffusion is equivalent in all directions; however, the human body is a complex structure divided into cells and extracellular compartments. The extracellular compartment, which contains water, exhibits free diffusion, whereas intracellular cells exhibit limited diffusion. Because of its complex structure and composition of axonal membranes and myelin sheath, human brain white matter exhibits anisotropic diffusion. As a result, diffusion in WM is anisotropic in nature [27]. Diffusion is an essential part of the human body's normal functioning, and unlike T1 and T2 relaxation times, which are affected by MRI parameters, diffusion is an intrinsic property that is independent of the MRI parameters used to measure it.

3.2.3 *b*-Factor

The term "*b*-value" or "*b*-factor" was coined derived from the landmark paper in 1965 by Stejskal and Tanner where they first introduced pulsed gradient diffusion method [28]. This technique is still followed by modern DWI pulse sequences which consist of two strong gradient pulses, separated by time as depicted in Fig. 3.2.

The sensitivity of any MRI pulse sequence is directly linked to the number of phase movements imposed by diffusion gradients. This movement is calculated using a parameter known as *b*-value or diffusion attenuation [29]. *b*-Value is a factor that depicts the strength and timing of the diffusion gradients used to map diffusion-weighted imaging.

b-Value depends mainly on three parameters: gradient interval, strength and duration. The main parameter which is altered in multiple *b*-values is gradient amplitude which is now used clinically. The unit used to represent *b*-value is seconds per square millimetre (s/mm^2). There are two extremes of *b*-values, i.e. high and low. The low value is 0 and the high value is in the range of 1000, but the typical range of values used in clinical diffusion weighting is 800–1500 s/mm^2. A low *b*-value is used with other *b*-values to calculate the apparent diffusion coefficient (ADC). In comparison with greater *b*-values, MR sequences with reduced *b*-values show images with greater SNR and reduced diffusion-weighted characteristics and the higher the *b*-value, the stronger the diffusion effects.

b-Value is an MR imaging parameter that is selected by the technologist before imaging. This directly controls the degree of diffusion weighting similar to choosing the time of echo (TE) which affects T2 weighting. Thus, diffusion is another relaxation mechanism in addition to T1 and T2. When we compare diffusion sequences with their counterpart pulse sequences, the relaxation mechanism affecting the final signal is less than 5%. However, when diffusion gradients are applied in DWI, it becomes the dominant mechanism of tissue contrast.

The *b*-value is determined by signal averages, predicted pathology and anatomic regions [30–33]. Figure 3.3 depicts an example with *b*-values of 0, 1000 and 3000 s/mm^2 that shows more diffusion weighting as the *b*-value increases, but at the expense of more noise in the image.

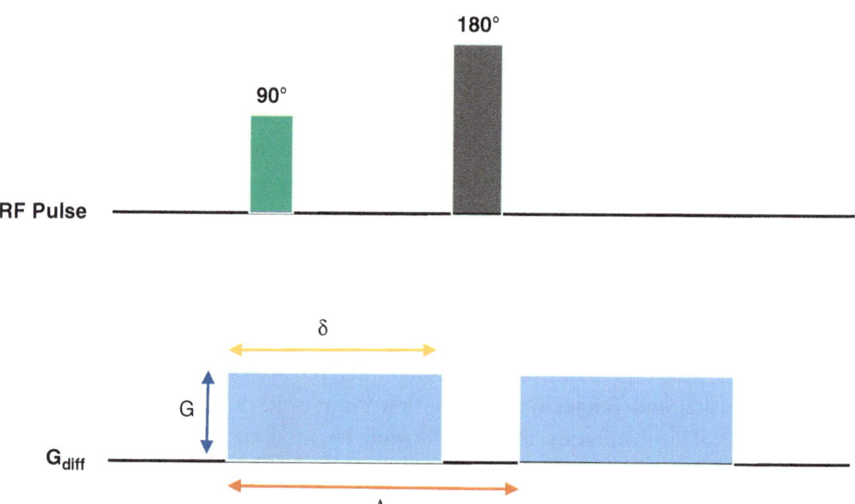

Fig. 3.2 Stejskal-Tanner pulsed diffusion gradient method

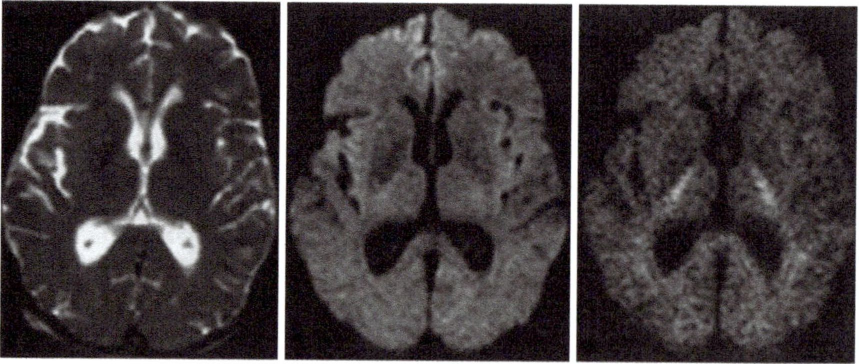

Fig. 3.3 Brain DWI with *b*-values of 0, 1000 and 3000 s/mm^2, respectively

3.2.4 Measurement of DWI: How Does Diffusion Affect the MR Signal?

Stejskal and Tanner proposed the MRI pulse sequences used for DWI in 1965 [28]. The basic technique involved the addition of diffusion gradients to probe molecular motion for measuring the MR signal. On both sides of a spin-echo pulse sequence's 180° refocusing RF pulse, two identical gradients with different polarities were used. The contrast mechanism, however, would be the same for both gradient schemes. The combination of these two events leads to the generation of a *b*-value. The higher the *b*-value, the more pronounced will be the diffusion-weighted signal. The first step to data extraction is to acquire a T2* image with no diffusion gradient which is $b = 0$. The next step is to access the diffusion of water in a minimum of three orthogonal directions as depicted in Fig. 3.4.

The entire process of DWI measurement can be explained with the help of stationary and moving water molecules. The application of the first gradient enables the stationary water molecules to acquire phase information. After the application of the 180-degree refocusing pulse, they are exposed to the same gradient which will cancel out the effects of the first. Hence they retain their original signal. On the other hand, moving water molecules acquire phase information by the first gradient followed by the second gradient as they are not in the same location due to continuous movement. Hence they are not rephased and lose their signal [20, 34, 35]. In the case of a brain infarct, the area affected by the stroke will be seen as a hyperintense area on the diffusion-weighted image and a hypointense area on the apparent diffusion coefficient (ADC) image.

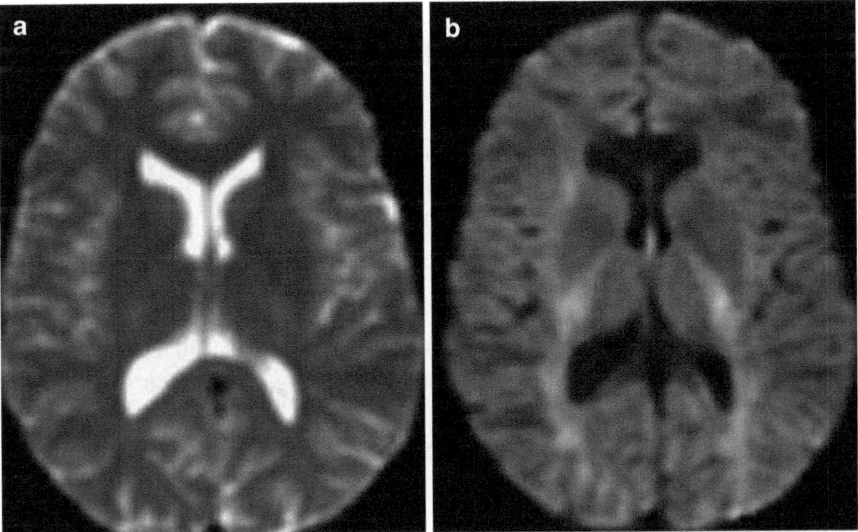

Fig. 3.4 (**a**) T2W image, (**b**) DWI image

3.2.5 DWI Image Contrast and ADC Calculation

Tissue permeability is very well demonstrated by its ability to diffuse through cell structure. This is calculated using the apparent diffusion coefficient. This parameter is not influenced by other extrinsic and intrinsic parameters that affect conventional MR imaging, and all these calculations are done using computer software. The speciality of ADC is that it appears exactly the reverse of DWI [36].

Diffusion gradients can be used to generate diffusion-weighted images, but the signal intensity and image contrast are dependent on the apparent diffusion coefficient (ADC). Because liquids have a high ADC, they appear bright or hyperintense. ADC must be calculated using at least two diffusion-weighted measurements with different *b*-values. As a result, by determining the signal intensity at the higher and lower *b*-values, the ADC can be calculated precisely. The mean signal intensities for each pixel in the region of interest are then used to generate an ADC map.

Image contrast in DWI can be confusing with a mix of different contrasts on display. Most of the DWI pulse sequences employ long echo times between 50 and 125 ms due to the prolonged diffusion process. As a result, diffusion-weighted images are referred to as T2 weighted images, and it can be difficult to distinguish between diffusion and T2 effects, as shown in Fig. 3.4. This effect, known as the T2 shine-through effect, causes a misrepresentation of normal anatomy and pathology in the brain MRIs [30, 37]. Another significant disadvantage of using long echo times is that diffusion-weighted images have a low signal-to-noise ratio. As a result, diffusion weighting reduces the signal from non-liquid tissues, resulting in low signal intensity on DWI. As a result, the majority of the newer MRI pulse sequences use signal intensity increasing techniques. ADC calculation can also be improved by lowering the signal-to-noise ratio at *b*-values greater than 1000 [38, 39].

3.2.6 Pulse Sequences Employed for DWI

When MRI was used in its early days for brain and body imaging, the random motion in DWI was considered as a spoiler to image quality because it affected SNR and caused artefacts. Water in its pure state exhibits isotropic diffusion and moves freely in all directions in an environment without restriction. A special quantity known as diffusion coefficient is used to define diffusion in restricted areas [40]. Spin-echo sequences are highly influenced by the diffusion effects which were discovered by Erwin Hahn [41]. Soon an algorithm was formed to describe phase shifts from the Larmor equation to calculate the diffusion coefficient [10]. Later, this algorithm was further modified which used similar gradients on both sides of the 180° radiofrequency pulses.

Gradients of diffusion sensitization are applied on either side of the 180° refocusing pulse in a DWI sequence, as shown in Fig. 3.5. The diffusion weighting of the image is influenced by the "*b*-value" parameter, and it is expressed in s/mm^2. The qualitative evaluation of diffusion is done using trace images, and the quantitative evaluation is done using the apparent diffusion coefficient (ADC). Tissues with

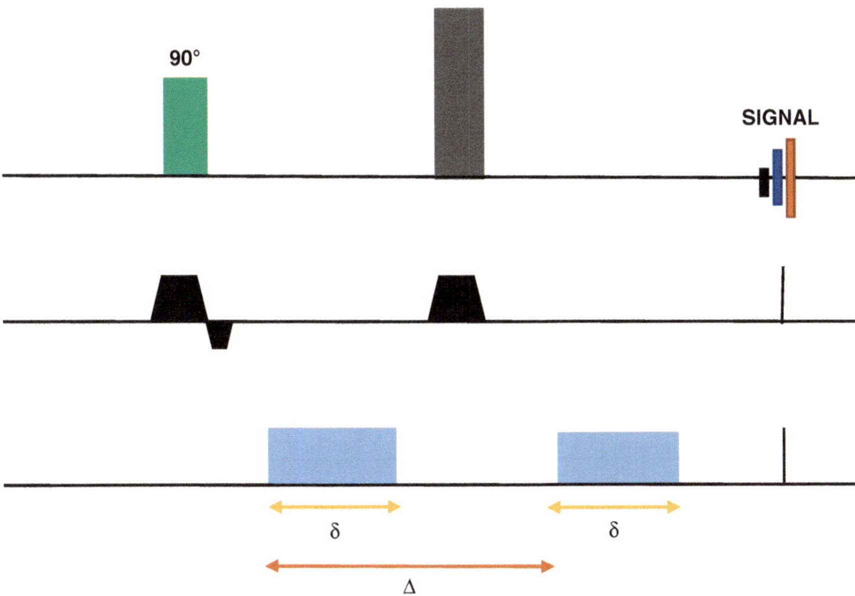

Fig. 3.5 DWI pulse sequence

restricted diffusion appear bright on the trace or DWI image and hypointense on the ADC map. For image acquisition, DWI employs a special fat-suppressed advanced echo-planar imaging [42]. Until the advent of EPI in the 1990s, DWI was ineffective in the field of imaging. Diffusion sequences based on EPI were faster and had fewer motion artefacts. The principle used in EPI is based on the technique of using time-sensitive fast encoding gradients instead of routine gradients used in conventional sequences. To improve SNR, advanced coils are used for imaging.

3.2.6.1 Echo-Planar Imaging in DWI-EPI Technical Overview

EPI is considered a superfast imaging technique because it uses either spin or gradient echo for an entire 2D image to be acquired in a single excitation or chain of echo train length and its k-space filling as depicted in Fig. 3.6. The advancements in gradient and spin-echo pulse sequences have led to the image acquisition in 50–90 ms with reduced motion artefacts. The roots of the discovery of EPI is considered as one of the oldest methods of spatial localization in MRI where the first biologic EPI images obtained were of a rabbit heart and an infant human heart in 1981 and 1983, respectively [43].

EPI is classified into two main types mainly the spin-echo EPI and gradient-echo EPI as shown in Figs. 3.7 and 3.8. Most recently we call them single-shot EPI and multi-shot EPI respectively as shown in Fig. 3.9. The echo train length, or shot facto, is the number of k-space rows in a single shot [44–48]. In the modern glossary, these are termed single-shot EPI and multi-shot EPI.

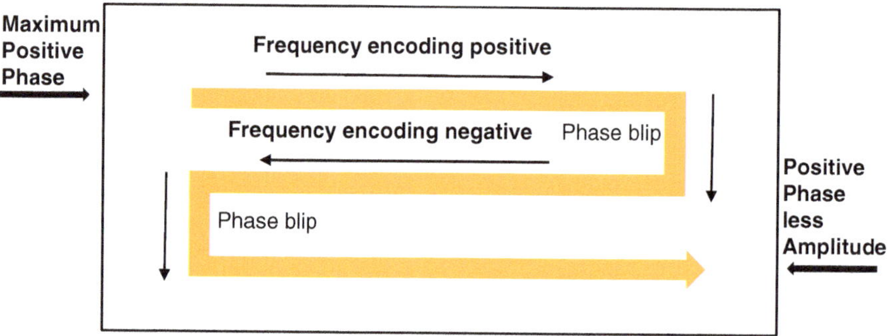

Fig. 3.6 k-space filling in EPI

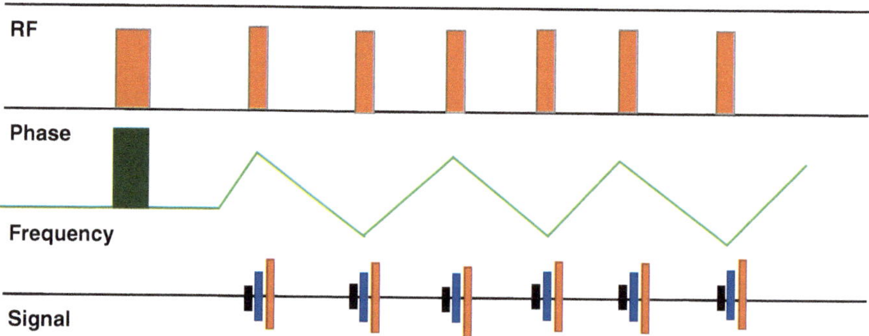

Fig. 3.7 GE-EPI

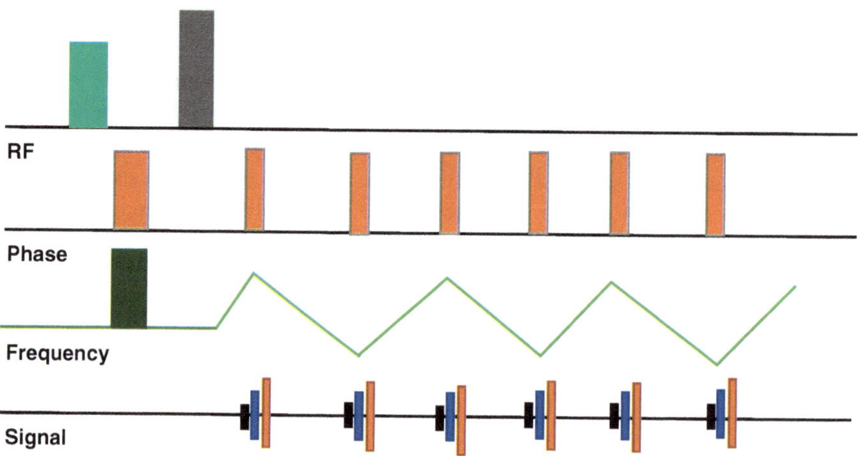

Fig. 3.8 SE-EPI

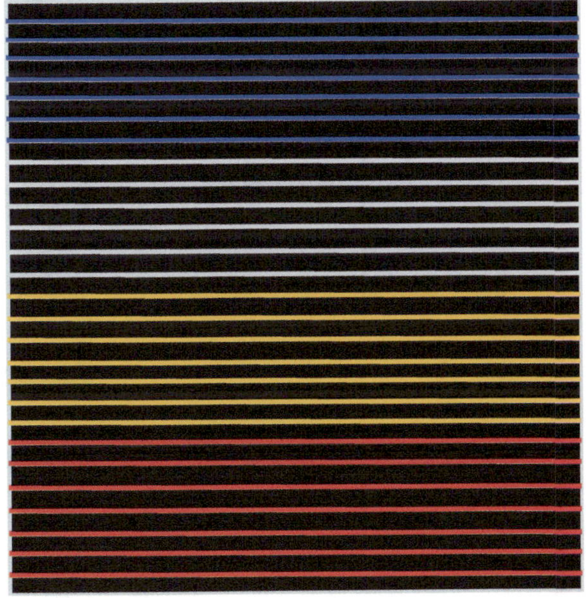

Fig. 3.9 Single- and multi-shot EPI

3.2.6.2 Parallel Imaging Technical Overview

Parallel imaging is an alternative technique superior to EPI in fast imaging. In this technique, k-space filling is more efficient, i.e. by filling multiple lines of k-space per TR, unlike other similar fast imaging techniques. To increase the speed of image acquisition, parallel imaging employs multiple coils and couples them together via software networking. As a result, the number of phase-encoding steps decreases, and thus the imaging time decreases [49, 50]. These coils have multiple channels as well, and typically the coil number ranges from 2 to 128 and so on as shown in Fig. 3.10.

DWI exhibits a low SNR especially in those anatomical areas that require high *b*-values (e.g. brain). There is absolutely no doubt that EPI is quick in data collection, but they still display a signal loss with low resolution after all the efforts made by advanced EPI sequences. EPI sequences also require a longer scan time to obtain extra data for mapping correction and motion reduction. These limitations can easily be tackled using parallel imaging techniques as it works with phased-array coils. The technology involves the use of faster gradient switching to reduce the overall scan time as shown in Fig. 3.11. The number of phase-encoding steps is manipulated by sampling incomplete k-space lines. However, parallel imaging techniques never alter the contrast characteristics. There are several parallel imaging techniques available in the imaging industry like SENSE, ASSET, GRAPPA and so on. These techniques are coupled with EPI techniques which acquire the same image data in lesser time without affecting contrast features [50–52].

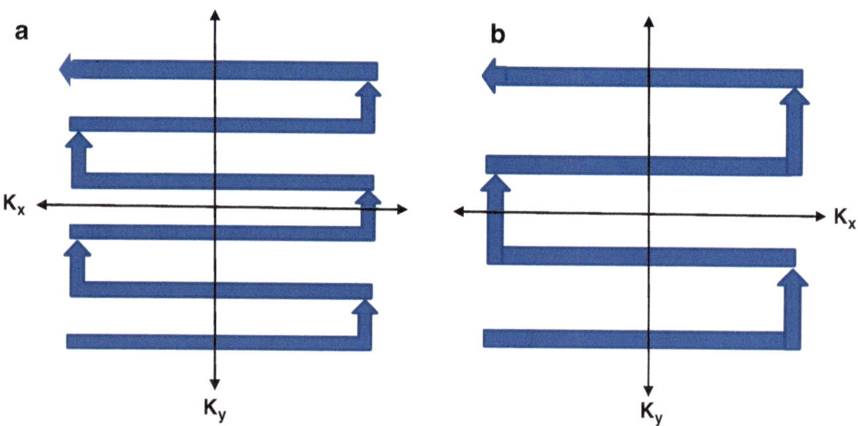

Fig. 3.10 Filling k-space by EPI. (**a**) Conventional vs. (**b**) parallel imaging

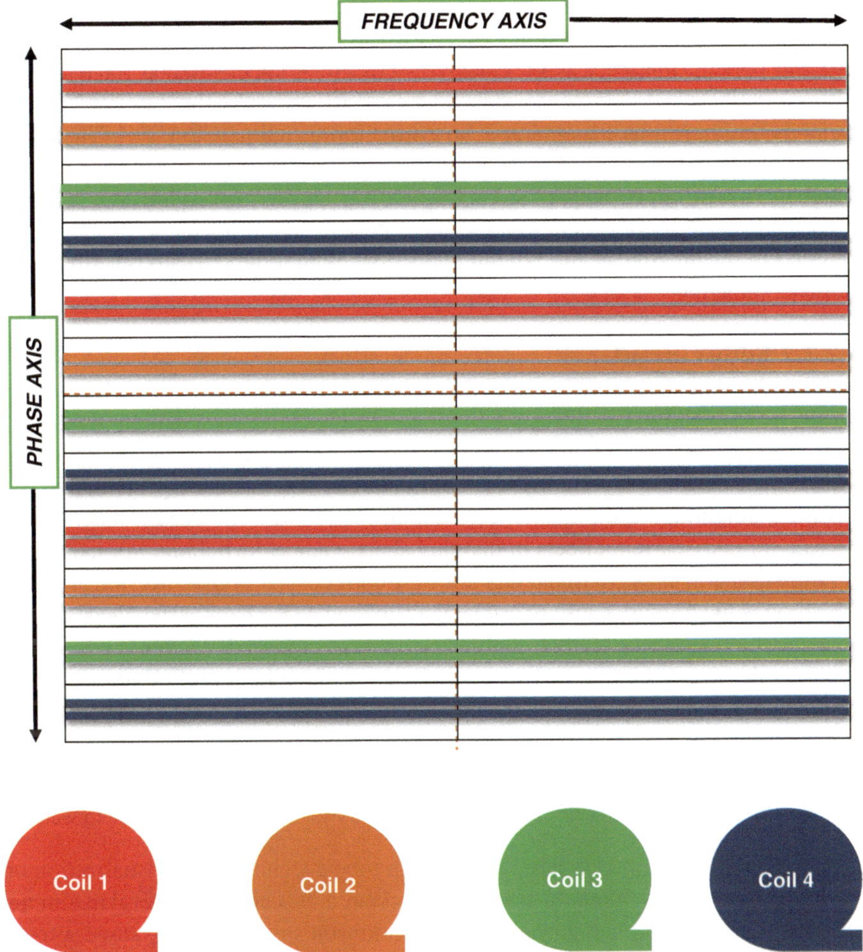

Fig. 3.11 Parallel imaging techniques

3.2.7 DWI Artefacts

3.2.7.1 Motion Artefacts

Motion sensitivity, as previously stated, is an undesirable effect in all diffusion-weighted imaging sequences [34]. The addition of diffusion gradients makes the pulse sequence sensitive to molecule motion, but it is also susceptible to micrometre-scale macroscopic motion. As a result, even minor and involuntary patient movements like cardiac, bowel, swallowing and breathing can cause image degradation due to motion artefacts, specifically ghosting in the phase-encoding direction. Several techniques have been proposed for reducing motion artefacts in diffusion-weighted imaging. The simplest way to reduce motion artefacts is to target the region being imaged while holding your breath or by using a cardiac gating [53] so that any kind of motion can be minimized. Another method for reducing motion is to shorten image acquisition times by employing fast imaging techniques such as EPI and parallel imaging, as previously discussed. Another method for reducing motion artefacts is to correct motion-related phase errors in the raw data. These methods are known as navigation echo correction techniques [54, 55]. There are several navigation techniques available, including spiral, self and auto navigated, which work with either radial or spiral k-space trajectories in every readout process. Advanced image reconstruction algorithms, in addition to navigation techniques, play a significant role in the overall reduction of motion artefacts in diffusion-weighted imaging.

3.2.7.2 Eddy Currents

Another disadvantage of diffusion-weighted imaging sequences is the eddy current caused by long and strong diffusion gradients used for image acquisition. Eddy currents are microelectric currents produced in coils by switching magnetic fields on and off. As a result of these currents, additional gradient fields are generated in the diffusion weighting, resulting in distorted images [27]. Most modern scanners compensate for eddy current effects in imaging short gradient switching; however, longer diffusion gradients are frequently not well-corrected [22, 56]. Diffusion gradient distortion is the primary cause of artefacts visible on ADC maps as enhanced edges. To avoid these artefacts, many techniques have been proposed, the most common of which is the use of bipolar diffusion gradients or the addition of additional 1800 pulses with the same or opposite polarity during the diffusion preparation [27].

3.2.8 DWI Applications

Diffusion-weighted imaging has emerged as a robust technique for visualization of the human brain, particularly in acute brain ischemia. It is also very useful in tumour characterization, acute and chronic stroke, Parkinson's disease, cyst, abscess from necrotic tumours, herpes, diffuse axonal imaging, gliomas, meningiomas, active demyelination, prostate lesions, otitis media, breast body and spine imaging [53, 57–68].

Summary: In this chapter, we have introduced the physics behind diffusion-weighted imaging. In Chap. 4, we shall be discussing the physics behind diffusion tensor imaging in detail.

References

1. Seidl AH. Regulation of conduction time along axons. Neuroscience. 2014;276:126–34.
2. Mitew S, Hay CM, Peckham H, Xiao J, Koenning M, Emery B. Mechanisms regulating the development of oligodendrocytes and central nervous system myelin. Neuroscience. 2014;276:29–47. https://www.sciencedirect.com/science/article/abs/pii/S0306452213009767?via%3Dihub.

3. Lundgaard I, Osório MJ, Kress B, Sanggaard S, Nedergaard M. White matter astrocytes in health and disease. 2013. http://europepmc.org/backend/ptpmcrender.fcgi?accid=PMC4016995&blobtype=pdf.
4. Bartzokis G. Neuroglialpharmacology: myelination as a shared mechanism of action of psychotropic treatments. Neuropharmacology. 2012;62(7):2137–53. https://linkinghub.elsevier.com/retrieve/pii/S0028390812000354.
5. Barkovich AJ. Concepts of myelin and myelination in neuroradiology. AJNR Am J Neuroradiol. 2000;21(6):1099–109. http://www.ncbi.nlm.nih.gov/pubmed/10871022.
6. Allen NJ, Barres BA. Neuroscience: glia—more than just brain glue. Nature. 2009;457(7230):675–7. http://www.ncbi.nlm.nih.gov/pubmed/19194443.
7. Singer JR. NMR diffusion and flow measurements and an introduction to spin phase graphing. J Phys E Sci Instrum. 1978;11(4):281.
8. Schlu M, Drescher R, Rexilius J, Lukas C, Hahn HK, Przuntek H, et al. Diffusion tensor imaging-based fractional anisotropy quantification in the corticospinal tract of patients with amyotrophic lateral. AJNR Am J Neuroradiol. 2007;28(4):724–30.
9. Rulseh AM, Keller J, Tintěra J, Kožíšek M, Vymazal J. Chasing shadows: what determines DTI metrics in gray matter regions? An in vitro and in vivo study. J Magn Reson Imaging. 2013;38(5):1103–10. http://doi.wiley.com/10.1002/jmri.24065.
10. Carr H, Purcell E. Effects of diffusion on free precession in nuclear magnetic resonance experiments. Phys Rev. 1954;94(3):630–8. http://link.aps.org/doi/10.1103/PhysRev.94.630.
11. Hrabe J, Kaur G, Guilfoyle DN. Principles and limitations of NMR diffusion measurements. J Med Phys. 2007;32(1):34–42. https://pubmed.ncbi.nlm.nih.gov/21217917.
12. Kuchel PW, Pagès G, Nagashima K, Velan S, Vijayaragavan V, Nagarajan V, et al. Stejskal-tanner equation derived in full. Concepts Magn Reson Part A Bridg Educ Res. 2012;40:A(5).
13. Sinnaeve D. The Stejskal-Tanner equation generalized for any gradient shape-an overview of most pulse sequences measuring free diffusion. Concepts Magn Reson Part A Bridg Educ Res. 2012;40:A(2).
14. Pierpaoli C, Basser PJ. Toward a quantitative assessment of diffusion anisotropy. Magn Reson Med. 1996;36(6):893–906. http://www.ncbi.nlm.nih.gov/pubmed/8946355.
15. Basser PJ, Pajevic S, Pierpaoli C, Duda J, Aldroubi A. In vivo fiber tractography using DT-MRI data. Magn Reson Med. 2000;44(4):625–32.
16. Koh DM, Collins DJ. Diffusion-weighted MRI in the body: applications and challenges in oncology. Am J Roentgenol. 2007;188(6):1622–35.
17. Padhani AR, Liu G, Mu-Koh D, Chenevert TL, Thoeny HC, Takahara T, et al. Diffusion-weighted magnetic resonance imaging as a cancer biomarker: consensus and recommendations. Neoplasia. 2009;11(2):102–25.
18. Heiervang E, Behrens TEJ, Mackay CE, Robson MD, Johansen-Berg H. Between session reproducibility and between subject variability of diffusion MR and tractography measures. Neuroimage. 2006;33(3):867–77. http://www.ncbi.nlm.nih.gov/pubmed/17000119.
19. Behrens TEJ, Woolrich MW, Jenkinson M, Johansen-Berg H, Nunes RG, Clare S, et al. Characterization and propagation of uncertainty in diffusion-weighted MR imaging. Magn Reson Med. 2003;50(5):1077–88.
20. Drake-Pérez M, Boto J, Fitsiori A, Lovblad K, Vargas MI. Clinical applications of diffusion weighted imaging in neuroradiology. Insights Imaging. 2018;9(4):535–47.
21. Edlow BL, Hurwitz S, Edlow JA. Diagnosis of DWI-negative acute ischemic stroke. Neurology. 2017;89(3):256–62.
22. Makin SDJ, Doubal FN, Dennis MS, Wardlaw JM. Clinically confirmed stroke with negative diffusion-weighted imaging magnetic resonance imaging: longitudinal study of clinical outcomes, stroke recurrence, and systematic review. Stroke. 2015;46(11):3142–8.
23. Uhlenbeck GE, Ornstein LS. On the theory of the Brownian motion. Phys Rev. 1930;36(5):823–41.
24. Caldeira AO, Leggett AJ. Path integral approach to quantum Brownian motion. Phys A Stat Mech Appl. 1983;121(3):587–616.

25. Einstein A. Über die von der molekularkinetischen Theorie der Wärme geforderte Bewegung von in ruhenden Flüssigkeiten suspendierten Teilchen. Ann Phys. 1905;322(8):549–60. http://doi.wiley.com/10.1002/andp.19053220806.
26. Fick's insight on liquid diffusion. [cited 2014 Jul 16]. http://www.olemiss.edu/sciencenet/saltnet/fick_insights_EOS.pdf.
27. Alexander AL, Lee JE, Lazar M, Field AS. Diffusion tensor imaging of the brain. Neurotherapeutics. 2007;4(3):316–29. http://www.ncbi.nlm.nih.gov/pubmed/17599699.
28. Stejskal EO, Tanner JE. Spin diffusion measurements: spin echoes in the presence of a time-dependent field gradient. J Chem Phys. 1965;42(1):288.
29. Bammer R, Holdsworth SJ, Veldhuis WB, Skare ST. New methods in diffusion-weighted and diffusion tensor imaging. Magn Reson Imaging Clin N Am. 2009;17(2):175–204. http://www.pubmedcentral.nih.gov/articlerender.fcgi?artid=2768271&tool=pmcentrez&rendertype=abstract.
30. Burdette JH, Durden DD, Elster AD, Yen YF. High b-value diffusion-weighted MRI of normal brain. J Comput Assist Tomogr. 2001;25(4):515–9. http://www.ncbi.nlm.nih.gov/pubmed/11473179.
31. Yoshiura T, Wu O, Zaheer A, Reese TG, Sorensen AG. Highly diffusion-sensitized MRI of brain: dissociation of gray and white matter. Magn Reson Med. 2001;45(5):734–40. http://www.ncbi.nlm.nih.gov/pubmed/11323798.
32. Pereira RS, Harris AD, Sevick RJ, Frayne R. Effect of b value on contrast during diffusion-weighted magnetic resonance imaging assessment of acute ischemic stroke. J Magn Reson Imaging. 2002;15(5):591–6. http://doi.wiley.com/10.1002/jmri.10105.
33. Kingsley PB, Monahan WG. Selection of the optimum b factor for diffusion-weighted magnetic resonance imaging assessment of ischemic stroke. Magn Reson Med. 2004;51(5):996–1001.
34. Bammer R. Basic principles of diffusion-weighted imaging. Eur J Radiol. 2003;45(3):169–84.
35. Fornasa F. Diffusion-weighted magnetic resonance imaging: what makes water run fast or slow? J Clin Imaging Sci. 2011;1(1):27.
36. Neil JJ. Diffusion imaging concepts for clinicians. J Magn Reson Imaging. 2008;27(1):1–7. http://www.ncbi.nlm.nih.gov/pubmed/18050325.
37. Chepuri NB, Yen Y, Burdette JH, Li H, Moody DM, Maldjian JA. Diffusion anisotropy in the corpus callosum. AJNR Am J Neuroradiol. 2002;23(5):803–8.
38. Lenglet C. Brain mapping. Amsterdam: Elsevier; 2015. p. 245–51. http://www.sciencedirect.com/science/article/pii/B9780123970251002918.
39. Shen J-M, Xia X-W, Kang W-G, Yuan J-J, Sheng L. The use of MRI apparent diffusion coefficient (ADC) in monitoring the development of brain infarction. BMC Med Imaging. 2011;11(1):2. http://www.pubmedcentral.nih.gov/articlerender.fcgi?artid=3022840&tool=pmcentrez&rendertype=abstract.
40. Beluffi G. Diffusion-weighted MR imaging. Applications in the body D.M. Koh H.C. Thoeni (Eds.). Radiol Med. 2011;116(3):499–500. http://link.springer.com/10.1007/s11547-011-0638-z.
41. Spin echoes. [cited 2014 Jul 15]. http://www.wmf.univ.szczecin.pl/~sergeev/Dydaktyka/Pr-R/Hahn-spin-echo.pdf.
42. Taouli B, Koh D-M. Diffusion-weighted MR imaging of the liver. Radiology. 2010;254(1):47–66. http://www.ncbi.nlm.nih.gov/pubmed/20032142.
43. Mansfield P. Multi-planar image formation using NMR spin echoes. J Phys C Solid State Phys. 1977;10(3):L55–8. http://stacks.iop.org/0022-3719/10/i=3/a=004?key=crossref.f48893f3d8bf21cb4a102c6293b5ce83.
44. Poustchi-Amin M, Mirowitz SA, Brown JJ, McKinstry RC, Li T. Principles and applications of echo-planar imaging: a review for the general radiologist. RadioGraphics. 2001;21(3):767–79. http://www.ncbi.nlm.nih.gov/pubmed/11353123.
45. Stehling MK, Turner R, Mansfield P. Echo-planar imaging: magnetic resonance imaging in a fraction of a second. Science. 1991;254(5028):43–50. http://www.ncbi.nlm.nih.gov/pubmed/1925560.

46. Hutter J, Price AN, Cordero-Grande L, Malik S, Ferrazzi G, Gaspar A, et al. Quiet echo planar imaging for functional and diffusion MRI. Magn Reson Med. 2018;79(3):1447–59.
47. Edelman RR, Wielopolski P, Schmitt F. Echo-planar MR imaging. Radiology. 1994;192(3):600–12.
48. Stehling MK, Schmitt F, Ladebeck R. Echo-planar MR imaging of human brain oxygenation changes. J Magn Reson Imaging. 1993;3(3):471–4.
49. Deshmane A, Gulani V, Griswold MA. HHS Public Access. 2015;36(1):55–72.
50. Schmiedeskamp H, Newbould RD, Pisani LJ, Skare S, Glover GH, Pruessmann KP, et al. Improvements in parallel imaging accelerated functional MRI using multiecho echo-planar imaging. Magn Reson Med. 2010;63(4):959–69.
51. Shen SH, Chiou YY, Wang JH, Yen MS, Lee RC, Lai CR, et al. Diffusion-weighted single-shot echo-planar imaging with parallel technique in assessment of endometrial cancer. Am J Roentgenol. 2008;190(2):481–8.
52. Hamilton J, Franson D, Seiberlich N. Recent advances in parallel imaging for MRI. Prog Nucl Magn Reson Spectrosc. 2017;101:71–95.
53. Le Bihan D, Douek P, Argyropoulou M, Turner R, Patronas N, Fulham M. Diffusion and perfusion magnetic resonance imaging in brain tumors. Top Magn Reson Imaging. 1993;5(1):25–31. http://www.ncbi.nlm.nih.gov/pubmed/8416686.
54. Mori S, Van Zijl PCM. A motion correction scheme by twin-echo navigation for diffusion-weighted magnetic resonance imaging with multiple RF echo acquisition. Magn Reson Med. 1998;40(4):511–6.
55. Taylor PA, Alhamud A, van der Kouwe A, Saleh MG, Laughton B, Meintjes E. Assessing the performance of different DTI motion correction strategies in the presence of EPI distortion correction. Hum Brain Mapp. 2016;37(12):4405–24.
56. Boelmans K, Bodammer NC, Suchorska B, Kaufmann J, Ebersbach G, Heinze HJ, et al. Diffusion tensor imaging of the corpus callosum differentiates corticobasal syndrome from Parkinson's disease. Park Relat Disord. 2010;16(8):498–502. https://doi.org/10.1016/j.parkreldis.2010.05.006.
57. Rordorf G, Koroshetz WJ, Copen WA, Cramer SC, Schaefer PW, Budzik RF, et al. Regional ischemia and ischemic injury in patients with acute middle cerebral artery stroke as defined by early diffusion-weighted and perfusion-weighted MRI. Stroke. 1998;29(5):939–43.
58. Rosenkrantz AB, Padhani AR, Chenevert TL, Koh DM, De Keyzer F, Taouli B, et al. Body diffusion kurtosis imaging: basic principles, applications, and considerations for clinical practice. J Magn Reson Imaging. 2015;42(5):1190–202.
59. Fisher M, Albers GW. Applications of diffusion-perfusion magnetic resonance imaging in acute ischemic stroke. Neurology. 1999;52(9):1750–6.
60. Sato K, Yuasa N, Fujita M, Fukushima Y. Clinical application of diffusion-weighted imaging for preoperative differentiation between uterine leiomyoma and leiomyosarcoma. Am J Obstet Gynecol. 2014;210(4):368.e1–8.
61. Kwee TC, Takahara T, Ochiai R, Katahira K, Van Cauteren M, Imai Y, et al. Whole-body diffusion-weighted magnetic resonance imaging. Eur J Radiol. 2009;70(3):409–17.
62. Roberts TPL, Rowley HA. Diffusion weighted magnetic resonance imaging in stroke. Eur J Radiol. 2003;45(3):185–94.
63. Thurnher MM, Law M. Diffusion-weighted imaging, diffusion-tensor imaging, and fiber tractography of the spinal cord. Magn Reson Imaging Clin N Am. 2009;17(2):225–44.
64. Vijithananda SM, Jayatilake ML, Weerakoon BS, Wathsala PGS, Thevapriya S, Thasanky S, et al. Skewness and kurtosis of apparent diffusion coefficient in human brain lesions to distinguish benign and malignant using MRI. In: Communications in computer and information science. Berlin: Springer; 2019.
65. Péran P, Cherubini A, Assogna F, Piras F, Quattrocchi C, Peppe A, et al. Magnetic resonance imaging markers of Parkinson's disease nigrostriatal signature. Brain. 2010;133(11):3423–33. http://www.ncbi.nlm.nih.gov/pubmed/20736190.
66. Kim CK, Jang SM, Park BK. Diffusion tensor imaging of normal prostate at 3T: effect of number of diffusion-encoding directions on quantitation and image quality. Br J Radiol.

2012;85(1015):e279–83. http://www.pubmedcentral.nih.gov/articlerender.fcgi?artid=3474052&tool=pmcentrez&rendertype=abstract.

67. Walhovd KB, Johansen-Berg H, Káradóttir RT. Unraveling the secrets of white matter—bridging the gap between cellular, animal and human imaging studies. Neuroscience. 2014;276:2–13. http://www.sciencedirect.com/science/article/pii/S0306452214005430.
68. Boll DT, Merkle EM. Diffuse liver disease: strategies for hepatic CT and MR imaging. Radiographics. 2009;29(6):1591–614. http://www.ncbi.nlm.nih.gov/pubmed/19959510.

Advanced MRI Neuroimaging Technique: Diffusion-Tensor Imaging

4

This chapter discusses the fundamental physics of water molecules' microstructural Brownian motion. The techniques related to diffusion-weighted imaging probe the movement of tissue microstructure which is reflected by its freedom of motion of water molecules. The apparent diffusion coefficient (ADC) maps are free from the effects of T1 and T2 relaxation. Diffusion-weighted imaging (DWI) gives us information on the restricted flow areas within the brain but does not give us its accurate length and direction. DTI, on the other hand, allows us to measure the length and direction of diffusion anisotropy in water molecules in real time. Parallel imaging and echo-planar imaging (EPI) techniques employing quick data acquisition with reduced artefacts are employed in DWI and DTI.

4.1 Introduction to Diffusion-Tensor Imaging (DTI)

The more advanced and sophisticated form of DWI which has already gained a lot of attention in recent times is diffusion-tensor imaging (DTI). As quoted previously, DWI provides both quantitative and qualitative information regarding properties of diffusion, and the addition of its functional component makes it the first choice of diagnosis in neuroimaging. Water diffusion in the brain's white matter is anisotropic because axon membranes limit the movement of molecules perpendicular to fibres. DTI uses this property to provide white-matter integrity data and to produce white-matter tract micro-architectural details.

R. P. Kotian, P. Koteshwar, *Diffusion Tensor Imaging and Fractional Anisotropy*,
https://doi.org/10.1007/978-981-19-5001-8_4

4.1.1 DTI Evolution

Depending on the spatial direction of the diffusion-encoding gradients, the white-matter contrast varies with the diffusion image [1]. The spatial direction concept, which stated that water diffusion in white-matter fibres was faster in one direction and slower in the opposite direction, i.e. anisotropic, was later justified and reported in the literature [2]. The initial attempts were very slow and non-progressive, as measurements for diffusion were done only along with two directions. Modern DTI came into being when tensor was used and 3D algorithms for fibre visualization were developed [3]. DTI's initial clinical uses were restricted to the central nervous system.

DTI is a new and advanced technique for imaging the brain white-matter fibres in vivo. Diffusion tensor along with functional MRI is gaining impetus in early diagnosis. With the help of this technique, diffusion anisotropy in tissue, the microstructure can be studied. DTI is one of the most sophisticated tools to measure water diffusion and tissue anisotropy [4]. A symmetric unit known as the diffusion tensor accurately measures the water diffusion [5]. More than six directions can be acquired to improve the accuracy of the diffusion-tensor estimation. As a result, there are two options: Increase the number of diffusion directions, or repeat the current diffusion-weighted directions.

4.2 Diffusion Anisotropy

Water diffusion in tissues is hampered by tissue structures such as cell organelles, macromolecules and cell membranes, as shown in Fig. 4.1, as opposed to free diffusion in pure water [6, 7]. These tissue obstacles cause collisions, which reduces the mean diffusion distance of water molecules, resulting in a lower diffusion coefficient known as apparent diffusion coefficient (ADC). ADC varies between tissues, owing primarily to the number and size of obstacles. The geometry of cell membranes, in addition to cell size and number, can cause variation in the ADC. The diffusion of water molecules, as shown in Fig. 4.1, can reflect an anisotropic arrangement of cells. Water flows more freely parallel to the cell's long axis than perpendicular to it. ADC measured perpendicular to cell orientation will therefore be less than ADC measured orthogonally. Anisotropy is the name given to this dependence property [5, 8].

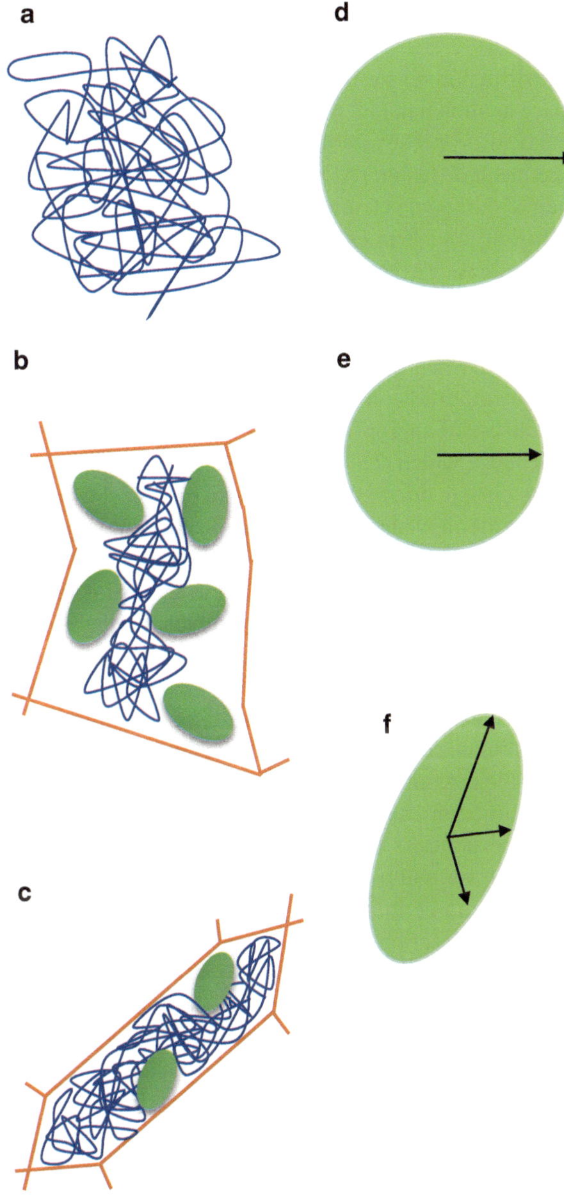

Fig. 4.1 Diffusion-tensor model. (**a**) Free diffusion in pure water. (**b**) Isotropic diffusion in tissue. (**c**) Anisotropic diffusion in tissue. (**d**) Free isotropic diffusion. (**e**) Hindered isotropic diffusion. (**f**) Hindered anisotropic diffusion in tissue

4.3 Diffusion-Tensor Matrix

The diffusion tensor is characterized by a 3 × 3 matrix to visualize diffusion in 3D space as shown in Fig. 4.2. An ellipsoid represents the diffusion tensor, and its mathematical properties allow its scalar measures to be extracted from tensor images. The mean diffusion (ADC), also known as the trace, is calculated by averaging the matrix's diagonal elements [9]. The principal direction is the direction of maximum diffusion, and it is calculated using the tensor's corresponding eigenvectors and eigenvalues. The eigenvalues describe the properties of the tensor, whereas the eigenvectors are orthogonal to each other. The eigenvalues are ranked as $\lambda 1 \geq \lambda 2 \geq \lambda 3$, and each corresponds to one eigenvector. The anisotropic diffusion is displayed when the eigenvalues differ from each other. When all eigenvalues are equivalent, diffusion is isotropic [10, 11] as shown in Fig. 4.1.

The use of appropriate field gradients in MRI affects the random motion of water molecules, which can be manipulated along the field gradient's direction. Diffusion is anisotropic due to the presence of myelin sheaths and axonal membranes, which restrict the movement of water molecules in white-matter fibre tracts. The orientation of the white-matter fibre tract corresponds to the direction of the maximum diffusivity [12]. This data is stored in the diffusion tensor, which is considered the real model of diffusion in a 3D structure. The diffusion tensor is a number matrix derived from several measurements of diffusion in various directions, from which the direction of maximum diffusivity can be precisely measured.

The tensor matrix is analogous to an ellipsoid with a diameter in each direction that estimates diffusivity in that direction. Figure 4.1 depicts the major axis oriented along the maximum diffusivity direction [4]. Because the degree of anisotropy and fibre direction can be mapped voxel by voxel, DTI can be used to study white-matter structures. The tensor model of diffusion is composed of a 3 × 3 matrix derived from multiple diffusivity measurements in at least six non-collinear directions, as shown in Fig. 4.3. Six diffusion-encoded measurements are needed to accurately describe the tensor, and increasing the number of directions improves tensor measurement accuracy [13–16]. The tensor matrix is diagonalized, yielding three eigenvectors describing the ellipsoid's major, medium and minor principal axes, which correspond to eigenvalues 1, 2 and 3 representing the apparent diffusivities along these axes, as shown in Fig. 4.3. When the shape of an ellipsoid

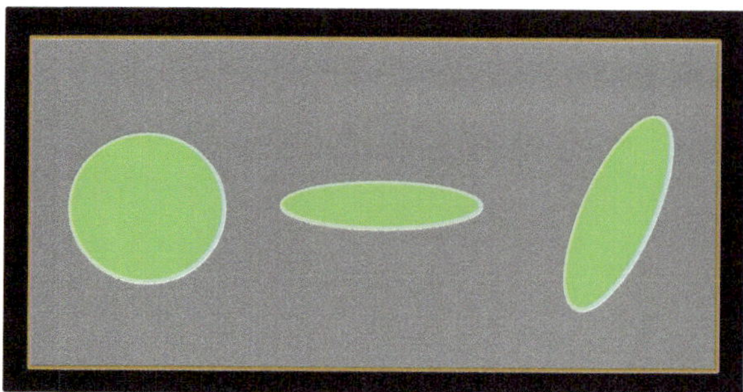

Fig. 4.2 Diffusion-tensor models (disc, sphere and elliptical)

Fig. 4.3 Tensor matrix

$$D_{isotropic} = \begin{bmatrix} D & 0 & 0 \\ 0 & D & 0 \\ 0 & 0 & D \end{bmatrix}$$

deviates from that of a sphere, the three tensor eigenvalues change and differ from one another, resulting in diffusion anisotropy. The available diffusivity measures are axial diffusivity, mean diffusivity, radial diffusivity and fractional anisotropy. The FA, which ranges from 0 to 1, is the most commonly used anisotropy metric. It is derived from the standard deviation of the three eigenvalues [17].

4.4 Trace Imaging

The Stejskal-Tanner imaging technique detected only molecular diffusion parallel to the diffusion gradient [18, 19]. Molecular motion perpendicular to the diffusion gradient, on the other hand, could not contribute to the final signal output. Protons in water molecules present in nerve fibres could freely move parallel to the fibre direction but not perpendicularly. This diffusion of spatial orientation was thus measured by implementing diffusion gradients in various spatial directions [7, 20]. Signal differences appeared in areas with high anisotropic diffusion, such as the corpus callosum. The corpus callosum showed decreased signals when the diffusion gradients were applied perpendicular to the nerve fibres, whereas it showed increased signals when the same gradients were applied parallel to the nerve fibres [21, 22]. ADC maps are created by combining average diffusivities of molecules in all spatial directions using three distinct direction-dependent maps. This measurement is also known as diffusion trace imaging because the direction-independent maps of tissue are directly proportional to the trace of the diffusion tensor [3, 23].

4.5 Measurement of Diffusion-Tensor Data

Diffusion anisotropy cannot be determined solely from three orthogonal diffusion measurements in any case. The measurements of a brain nerve fibre that runs diagonally across all three coordinate axes are identical to isotropic diffusion and cannot be distinguished. As a result, rigorous methods for obtaining data from anisotropic nerve fibres within the brain for diffusion-tensor evaluation are used. To obtain information from the full diffusion tensor and measure anisotropic diffusion, a minimum of six independent diffusion measurements are required [5]. Diffusion is measured using a tensor matrix with six independent components. As explained previously, each measurement is based on images with at least two different *b*-values. A *b*-value of 0 is used as a direction-independent reference for diffusion-tensor calculations [17]. As a result, no separate reference images for each diffusion direction are required. A typical DTI protocol includes one measurement without any diffusion weighting and a *b*-value of 0 and at least six diffusion-weighted measurements with different gradient directions. To capture all necessary data, these gradient directions should be "as diverse as possible". An ideal DTI *b*-value for brain imaging is 1000 s/mm^2, with a range of 800–1200 s/mm^2 [24, 25].

The best way to visualize diffusion-tensor information about tissue microstructure is with a three-dimensional ellipsoid. In contrast, a single ellipsoid cannot describe the complex crossing of white-matter fibres in the brain. To overcome this limitation and provide accurate diffusion-tensor measurements, complex techniques like high-angular resolution imaging, q-ball imaging and diffusion kurtosis have been developed [26–30].

4.6 Anisotropy Indices

Anisotropy indices are considered rotationally invariant and are formed by the eigenvalues of the tensor [3]. However, this relationship between the eigenvalues reflects the true characteristics of diffusion. Diffusion tensors can be calculated, and their scalar measurements can be derived using multiple image processing tools. FA is the most commonly used DTI-derived fibre integrity metric [31–33]. It shows the normal integrity of neuronal fibre tracts with myelination. The diameter and density of the fibre can be accurately computed using FA. FA is calculated from the tensor eigenvalues ($\lambda 1$, $\lambda 2$, $\lambda 3$). The shape of diffusion using its scalar derivative is thus derived by its fractional anisotropy. Finally, FA is validated by measuring its eigenvalue to the mean of all eigenvalues, as shown in the equation below. The visualization of diffusion-tensor data over an imaging slice is very difficult; hence, colour-coded maps are used to display FA values or maps. In the colour-coded maps, red corresponds to diffusion along the x-axis (inferior superior), blue to diffusion along the y-axis (transverse axis) and green to diffusion along the z-axis (anterior-posterior). However, the intensity of the colour is directly proportional to the signal of the fractional anisotropy as depicted in Fig. 4.4.

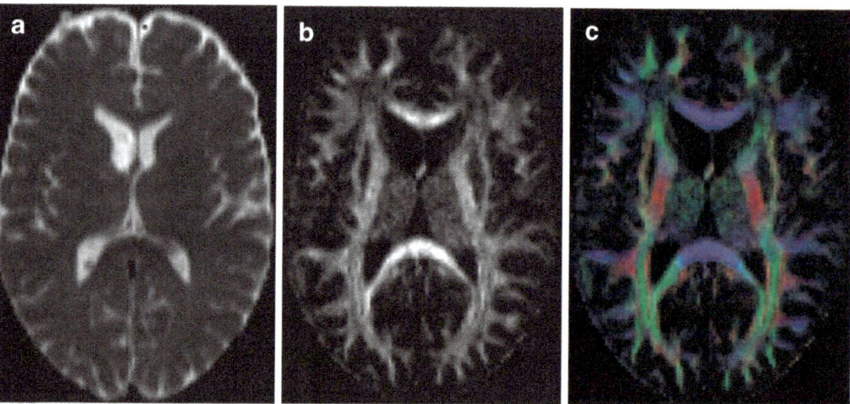

Fig. 4.4 (**a**) ADC. (**b**) FA and (**c**) color-coded FA images

The mean diffusivity (MD), radial diffusivity (RD) and axial diffusivity (AD) are the other diffusion derivatives. Individual parallel and perpendicular diffusivity measures are essential for the interpretation of FA and MD values, and their related abnormalities since anisotropy can be decreased owing to a reduction in parallel or an increase in perpendicular diffusivity or a mixture of both.

Axial or parallel diffusivity (AD) represents the principal eigenvalue ($\lambda 1$) of the diffusion tensor—that is, the dominant diffusion direction within the voxel (i.e. along with the dominant fibre) as shown in Fig. 4.5. AD has been linked with axonal integrity. AD represents diffusion parallel to the axon axis.

4.6.1 Radial or Perpendicular Diffusivity (RD)

The other two eigenvalues of the tensor (($\lambda 2$, $\lambda 3$),) are characterized by radial or perpendicular diffusivity (RD), which measures diffusivity along two axes orthogonal to the principal one as depicted in Fig. 4.5. The average diffusivity value perpendicular to the axon is RD [34, 35].

$$FA = \frac{\sqrt{(\lambda 1-\lambda 2)^2+(\lambda 2-\lambda 3)^2+(\lambda 1-\lambda 3)^2}}{\sqrt{2(\lambda 1^2+\lambda 2^2+\lambda 3^2)}}$$

$$FA = \sqrt{\frac{3}{2}}\,\frac{\sqrt{(\lambda_1-(\lambda))^2+(\lambda_2-(\lambda))^2+(\lambda_3-(\lambda))^2}}{\sqrt{\lambda_1^2+\lambda_2^2+\lambda_3^2}}$$

And

$$RA = \sqrt{\frac{1}{3}}\,\frac{\sqrt{(\lambda_1-(\lambda))^2+(\lambda_2-(\lambda))^2+(\lambda_3-(\lambda))^2}}{(\lambda)}$$

Where,

$$(\lambda) = \frac{1}{3}(\lambda_1+\lambda_2+\lambda_3)$$

where,

FA = Fractional anisotropy values

$\lambda 1$, $\lambda 2$, $\lambda 3$ = eigen values

λ = Mean Diffusivity

(Mean diffusivity or ADC) = ($\lambda 1 + \lambda 2 + \lambda 3/3$)

&

where $\lambda 1$, $\lambda 2$ and $\lambda 3$ are the largest, intermediate and smallest eigenvalues respectively, of the diffusion

Fig. 4.5 FA, RA and ADC (MD) formulae

4.6.2 Mean Diffusivity (MD)

Mean diffusivity is the average of the three diagonal elements of the diffusion tensor as shown in Fig. 4.5. Mean diffusivity (MD) is a broad overview of diffusion measurements in all directions, within a voxel or area. It can be thought of as the average displacement of water molecules within the voxel. The presence of a visible impediment can be depicted very well using MD measurements:

$$D = \lambda 1 + \lambda 2 + \lambda 3 / 3$$

where D = mean diffusivity and $\lambda 1$, $\lambda 2$ and $\lambda 3$ = eigenvalues.

4.7 DTI Applications

DTI is a very powerful tool to give a thorough insight into the brain white matter through tractography. The current pitfalls in DTI are reduced signal-to-noise ratio and increased artefacts. Hence, new methods for image processing need to be processed to tackle these artefacts. Other limitations are as follows:

1. Wrong calculation of diffusion characteristics
2. Poor-quality tensors used in atlas building
3. Unknown influence of it in atlas building
4. Reliability of conclusions based on these data
5. FA value errors

Despite the above-mentioned pitfalls, DTI still finds numerous clinical applications in medicine. DTI's primary capability is to measure the motility of water molecules in tissue. Its peculiar characteristics demonstrate the exact orientation of the diffusion characteristics of white-matter tracts. The main clinical application of diffusion-tensor imaging lies within the central nervous system. However, its use for estimating anisotropy in the detection of certain pathologies is gaining impetus in recent times. DTI also claims to provide valuable information on diseases such as Parkinson's disease (PD), Alzheimer's disease (AD), epilepsy, ischemic stroke, traumatic brain injury, depression, spinal cord injuries, schizophrenia, multiple sclerosis, musculoskeletal and peripheral nerve pathology, focal cortical dysplasia, white-matter tumours and so on [31, 36–48].

Summary: In this chapter, we have introduced the image contrast mechanisms in T1-, T2- and PD-weighted images followed by DWI and DTI. In Chap. 5, we shall be discussing the primary scalar derivative of DTI, the fractional anisotropy, in detail.

References

1. Hunsche S, Moseley ME, Stoeter P, Hedehus M. Diffusion-tensor MR imaging at 1.5 and 3.0 T: initial observations. Radiology. 2001;221(2):550–6. http://pubs.rsna.org/doi/abs/10.1148/radiol.2212001823.
2. Le Bihan D, Douek P, Argyropoulou M, Turner R, Patronas N, Fulham M. Diffusion and perfusion magnetic resonance imaging in brain tumors. Top Magn Reson Imaging. 1993;5(1):25–31. http://www.ncbi.nlm.nih.gov/pubmed/8416686.
3. Pierpaoli C, Jezzard P, Basser PJ, Barnett A, Di Chiro G. Diffusion tensor MR imaging of the human brain. Radiology. 1996;201(3):637–48. http://www.ncbi.nlm.nih.gov/pubmed/8939209.
4. Basser PJ, Mattiello J, LeBihan D. MR diffusion tensor spectroscopy and imaging. Biophys J. 1994;66(1):259–67. http://www.pubmedcentral.nih.gov/articlerender.fcgi?artid=1275686&tool=pmcentrez&rendertype=abstract.
5. Basser PJ, Jones DK. Diffusion-tensor MRI: theory, experimental design and data analysis—a technical review. NMR Biomed. 2002;15(7–8):456–67. http://www.ncbi.nlm.nih.gov/pubmed/12489095.
6. Abdallah CG, Tang CY, Mathew SJ, Martinez J, Hof PR, Perera TD, et al. Diffusion tensor imaging in studying white matter complexity: a gap junction hypothesis. Neurosci Lett. 2010;475(3):161–4. http://www.sciencedirect.com/science/article/pii/S0304394010003915.
7. Liu Z, Farzinfar M, Katz LM, Zhu H, Goodlett CB, Gerig G, et al. Automated voxel-wise brain DTI analysis of fitness and aging. Open Med Imaging J. 2012;6(1):80–8.
8. Jun Q, Irvin Y, Paolo T, Yi M, Carissa S, Kang K. Tracking cerebral white matter changes across the lifespan: insights from diffusion tensor imaging studies. J Neural Transm (Vienna). 2013;120(9):1369–95.
9. Le Bihan D, Mangin JF, Poupon C, Clark CA, Pappata S, Molko N, et al. Diffusion tensor imaging: concepts and applications. J Magn Reson Imaging. 2001;13(4):534–46.
10. Pinheiro GR, Soares GS, Costa AL, Lotufo RA, Rittner L. Divergence map from diffusion tensor imaging: concepts and application to corpus callosum. In: Proceedings of the annual international conference of the IEEE Engineering in Medicine and Biology Society, EMBS; 2016.
11. Hagmann P, Jonasson L, Maeder P, Thiran J, Wedeen VJ, Meuli R. CENTRAL NERVOUS SYSTEM: STATE OF THE ART. Understanding diffusion MR imaging techniques: from scalar imaging to diffusion. RadioGraphics. 2006;26:205–24.
12. Moseley ME, Cohen Y, Kucharczyk J, Mintorovitch J, Asgari HS, Wendland MF, et al. Diffusion-weighted MR imaging of anisotropic water diffusion in cat central nervous system. Radiology. 1990;176(2):439–45. http://pubs.rsna.org/doi/10.1148/radiology.176.2.2367658.
13. Papadakis NG, Murrills CD, Hall LD, Huang CL, Adrian CT. Minimal gradient encoding for robust estimation of diffusion anisotropy. Magn Reson Imaging. 2000;18(6):671–9. http://www.ncbi.nlm.nih.gov/pubmed/10930776.
14. Hasan KM, Gupta RK, Santos RM, Wolinsky JS, Narayana PA. Diffusion tensor fractional anisotropy of the normal-appearing seven segments of the corpus callosum in healthy adults and relapsing-remitting multiple sclerosis patients. J Magn Reson Imaging. 2005;21(6):735–43. http://www.ncbi.nlm.nih.gov/pubmed/15906348.
15. Hasan KM, Parker DL, Alexander AL. Comparison of gradient encoding schemes for diffusion-tensor MRI. J Magn Reson Imaging. 2001;13(5):769–80. http://www.ncbi.nlm.nih.gov/pubmed/11329200.
16. Jones DK, Horsfield MA, Simmons A. Optimal strategies for measuring diffusion in anisotropic systems by magnetic resonance imaging. Magn Reson Med. 1999;42(3):515–25. http://www.ncbi.nlm.nih.gov/pubmed/10467296.
17. Pierpaoli C, Basser PJ. Toward a quantitative assessment of diffusion anisotropy. Magn Reson Med. 1996;36(6):893–906. http://www.ncbi.nlm.nih.gov/pubmed/8946355.
18. Stejskal EO, Tanner JE. Spin diffusion measurements: spin echoes in the presence of a time-dependent field gradient. J Chem Phys. 1965;42(1):288–92.

19. Sinnaeve D. The Stejskal-Tanner equation generalized for any gradient shape—an overview of most pulse sequences measuring free diffusion. Concepts Magn Reson Part A Bridg Educ Res. 2012;40:A(2).
20. Haakma W, Dik P, ten Haken B, Froeling M, Nievelstein RAJ, Cuppen I, et al. Diffusion tensor magnetic resonance imaging and fiber tractography of the sacral plexus in children with spina bifida. J Urol. 2014;192(3):927–33. http://www.sciencedirect.com/science/article/pii/S002253471403417X.
21. Sullivan EV, Rohlfing T, Pfefferbaum A. Longitudinal study of callosal microstructure in the normal adult aging brain using quantitative DTI fiber tracking. Dev Neuropsychol. 2010;35(3):233–56. http://www.pubmedcentral.nih.gov/articlerender.fcgi?artid=2867078&tool=pmcentrez&rendertype=abstract.
22. Genc S, Malpas CB, Ball G, Silk TJ, Seal ML. Age, sex, and puberty related development of the corpus callosum: a multi-technique diffusion MRI study. Brain Struct Funct. 2018;223(6):2753–65. http://www.ncbi.nlm.nih.gov/pubmed/29623479.
23. Melhem ER, Itoh R, Jones L, Barker PB. Diffusion tensor MR imaging of the brain: effect of diffusion weighting on trace and anisotropy measurements. AJNR Am J Neuroradiol. 2000;21(10):1813–20.
24. Chou M, Mori S. Effects of b-value and echo time on magnetic resonance diffusion tensor imaging-derived parameters at 1.5 T : a voxel-wise study. J Med Biol Eng. 2012;33(1):45–50.
25. Bisdas S, Bohning DEE, Besenski N, Nicholas JSS, Rumboldt Z. Reproducibility, interrater agreement, and age-related changes of fractional anisotropy measures at 3T in healthy subjects: effect of the applied b-value. AJNR Am J Neuroradiol. 2008;29(6):1128–33. http://www.ajnr.org/cgi/doi/10.3174/ajnr.A1044.
26. Caiazzo G, Trojsi F, Cirillo M, Tedeschi G, Esposito F. Q-ball imaging models: comparison between high and low angular resolution diffusion-weighted MRI protocols for investigation of brain white matter integrity. Neuroradiology. 2015;58:209–15. http://www.ncbi.nlm.nih.gov/pubmed/26573606.
27. Landgraf P, Merhof D, Richter M. Anisotropy of HARDI diffusion profiles based on the L2-norm. In: Bildverarbeitung für die Medizin. Berlin: Springer; 2011.
28. Lanzafame S, Giannelli M, Garaci F, Floris R, Duggento A, Guerrisi M, et al. Differences in Gaussian diffusion tensor imaging and non-Gaussian diffusion kurtosis imaging model-based estimates of diffusion tensor invariants in the human brain. Med Phys. 2016;43(5):2464. http://www.ncbi.nlm.nih.gov/pubmed/27147357.
29. Vijithananda SM, Jayatilake ML, Weerakoon BS, Wathsala PGS, Thevapriya S, Thasanky S, et al. Skewness and kurtosis of apparent diffusion coefficient in human brain lesions to distinguish benign and malignant using MRI, Communications in computer and information science. Berlin: Springer; 2019.
30. Steven AJ. Diffusion kurtosis imaging: environment of the brain. 2014;26–33.
31. Lerner A, Mogensen MA, Kim PE, Shiroishi MS, Hwang DH, Law M. Clinical applications of diffusion tensor imaging. World Neurosurg. 2014;82:96–109. http://deepblue.lib.umich.edu/bitstream/handle/2027.42/35153/1042?sequence=1.
32. Kingsley PB. Introduction to diffusion tensor imaging mathematics: part II. Anisotropy, diffusion-weighting factors, and gradient encoding schemes. Concepts Magn Reson Part A. 2006;28A(2):123–54.
33. Paper O. Normal development of human brain white matter from infancy to early adulthood: a diffusion tensor imaging study. Dev Neurosci. 2015;37(2):182–94.
34. Assaf Y, Pasternak O. Diffusion tensor imaging (DTI)-based white matter mapping in brain research: a review. J Mol Neurosci. 2008;34(1):51–61. http://www.ncbi.nlm.nih.gov/pubmed/18157658.
35. Assaf Y. Can we use diffusion MRI as a bio-marker of neurodegenerative processes? BioEssays. 2008;30(11–12):1235–45. http://www.ncbi.nlm.nih.gov/pubmed/18937377.

36. Ito M, Watanabe H, Kawai Y, Atsuta N, Tanaka F, Naganawa S, et al. Usefulness of combined fractional anisotropy and apparent diffusion coefficient values for detection of involvement in multiple system atrophy. J Neurol Neurosurg Psychiatry. 2007;78(7):722–8. http://www.pubmedcentral.nih.gov/articlerender.fcgi?artid=2117692&tool=pmcentrez&rendertype=abstract
37. Tae WS, Ham BJ, Pyun SB, Kang SH, Kim BJ. Current clinical applications of diffusion-tensor imaging in neurological disorders. J Clin Neurol (Korea). 2018;14(2):129–40.
38. Kim M, Park H. Using tractography to distinguish SWEDD from Parkinson's disease patients based on connectivity. Parkinsons Dis. 2016;2016:8704910.
39. Aquino D, Contarino V, Albanese A, Minati L, Farina L, Grisoli M, et al. Substantia nigra in Parkinson's disease: a multimodal MRI comparison between early and advanced stages of the disease. Neurol Sci. 2014;35(5):753–8.
40. Boelmans K, Christian N, Suchorska B, Kaufmann J, Ebersbach G, Heinze H, et al. Parkinsonism and related disorders diffusion tensor imaging of the corpus callosum differentiates corticobasal syndrome from Parkinson's disease q. Parkinsonism Relat Disord. 2017;16(8):498–502. https://doi.org/10.1016/j.parkreldis.2010.05.006.
41. Wiltshire K, Concha L, Gee M, Bouchard T, Beaulieu C, Camicioli R. Corpus callosum and cingulum tractography in Parkinson's disease. Can J Neurol Sci. 2010;37(5):595–600. http://www.ncbi.nlm.nih.gov/pubmed/21059504.
42. Péran P, Cherubini A, Assogna F, Piras F, Quattrocchi C, Peppe A, et al. Magnetic resonance imaging markers of Parkinson's disease nigrostriatal signature. Brain. 2010;133(11):3423–33. http://www.ncbi.nlm.nih.gov/pubmed/20736190.
43. Farrell JA, Landman BA, Jones CK, Smith SA, Prince JL, Van ZPC, et al. Effects of diffusion weighting scheme and SNR on DTI-derived fractional anisotropy at 1.5T introduction. Proc Intl Soc Mag Reson Med. 2006;993:2000.
44. Cascio CJ, Gerig G, Piven J. Diffusion tensor imaging: application to the study of the developing brain. J Am Acad Child Adolesc Psychiatry. 2007;46(2):213–23.
45. Costabile JD, Alaswad E, D'Souza S, Thompson JA, Ormond DR. Current applications of diffusion tensor imaging and tractography in intracranial tumor resection. Front Oncol. 2019;9:426.
46. Mukherjee P, Berman JI, Chung SW, Hess CP, Henry RG. Diffusion tensor MR imaging and fiber tractography: theoretic underpinnings. Am J Neuroradiol. 2008;29(4):632–41.
47. Clark CA, Werring DJ. Diffusion tensor imaging in spinal cord: Methods and applications—a review. NMR Biomed. 2002;15(7-8):578–86.
48. Kubicki M, Westin CF, Maier SE, Mamata H, Frumin M, Ersner-Hershfield H, et al. Diffusion tensor imaging and its application to neuropsychiatric disorders. Harv Rev Psychiatry. 2002;10(6):324–36.

Fractional Anisotropy: Scalar Derivative of Diffusion-Tensor Imaging

5

The previous chapter briefly described the physics behind diffusion anisotropy and diffusion-tensor imaging. The current chapter throws light on the most important scalar derivative of DTI, i.e. fractional anisotropy and its clinical utility on the brain white matter. The evidence on factors affecting FA values and normative FA have been outlined in-depth as well.

5.1 Introduction and Overview of Fractional Anisotropy (FA)

FA is used to express in vivo water diffusion that occurs in all directions. This value is a derivative and is one of the DTI scalar diffusivity measures. The DTI data serve as foundation for calculating eigenvectors and eigenvalues. Many parameters derived from eigenvectors are thus used for anisotropy quantification. Clinical trials conducted on these indices showed that FA demonstrates the degree of deviation from uniform diffusion very precisely [1] and provides the best performance in terms of image quality and resolution [2, 3].

FA is currently the best technique for measuring diffusion anisotropy and is extensively used in fibre tracking [1, 4]. Based on eigenvalues, FA is calculated mathematically using the following formulae where $\lambda 1$ represents the principal eigenvalue parallel to the axonal axis and $\lambda 2$, $\lambda 3$ characterizes eigenvalues perpendicular to the principal axon axis as depicted in Fig. 5.1.

where

FA = fractional anisotropy values
$\lambda 1, \lambda 2, \lambda 3$ = eigenvalues
λ = mean diffusivity
(mean diffusivity or ADC) = $(\lambda 1 + \lambda 2 + \lambda 3/3)$
and

R. P. Kotian, P. Koteshwar, *Diffusion Tensor Imaging and Fractional Anisotropy*, https://doi.org/10.1007/978-981-19-5001-8_5

where $\lambda 1$, $\lambda 2$ and $\lambda 3$ are the largest, intermediate and smallest eigenvalues, respectively, of the diffusion tensor [1, 5, 6].

A piece of detailed and age-specific knowledge regarding various white matter microstructures in the brain along with the regional and normal variation of FA values is very important for treatment and diagnosis in clinical cases where DTI measurements.

DTI is the only imaging technique that can detect water diffusion in the brain. DTI, an imaging technique that is extremely sensitive to water diffusion in the brain, is the only way to see it. Isotropic diffusion is diffusion that occurs equally in all directions, whereas anisotropic diffusion is diffusion that is restricted by a barrier.

FA is the diffusion parameter obtained from DTI [7]. FA is a scalar diffusion directionality parameter that has a value between 0 and 1. FA, a scaler quantity ranging from 0 to 1, represents diffusion directionality, with 0 representing completely isotropic diffusion and 1 representing highly anisotropic diffusion, as shown in Fig. 5.2. An example of a color-coded FA map is shown in Fig. 5.3. Despite the extensive use of DTI techniques, only a few studies have examined normative FA values [8–19].

Fig. 5.1 FA value calculation formulae

$$FA = \sqrt{\frac{3}{2}} \frac{\sqrt{(\lambda_1 - (\lambda))^2 + (\lambda_2 - (\lambda))^2 + (\lambda_3 - (\lambda))^2}}{\sqrt{(\lambda 1^2 + \lambda 2^2 + \lambda 3^2)}}$$

$$(\lambda) = \frac{1}{3}(\lambda_1 + \lambda_2 + \lambda_3)$$

$$FA = \frac{\sqrt{(\lambda 1 - \lambda 2)^2 + (\lambda 2 - \lambda 3)^2 + (\lambda 1 - \lambda 3)^2}}{\sqrt{2(\lambda 1^2 + \lambda 2^2 + \lambda 3^2)}}$$

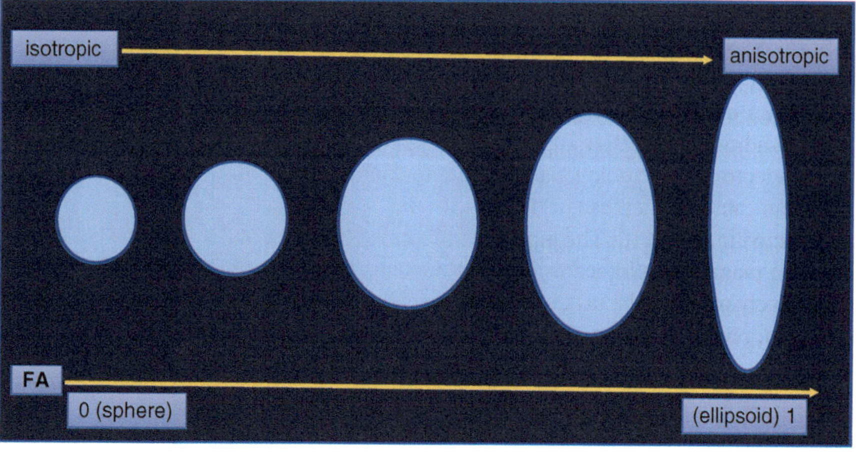

Fig. 5.2 FA range between 0 and 1

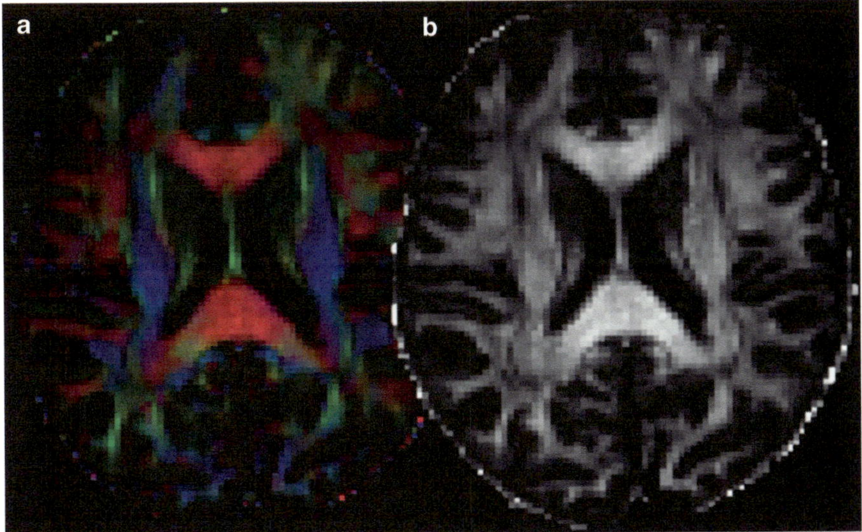

Fig. 5.3 (**a**) Color-coded FA maps; (**b**) diffusion-weighted image

Fibres with left-right orientation are encoded in red, with inferior-superior orientation in blue and those with anterior-posterior direction in green. FA provides important information about microstructural white matter (WM) substrate; it is non-specific reflecting fibre orientation, dispersion, neuronal density, axonal diameter and myelination degree.

FA has enough sensitivity to characterize various pathological brain conditions and also represents a robust DTI measurement. The complexity of WM configuration might also result in a particular situation when FA does not change much, whereas diffusivity values may vary especially if water diffusion increases in all directions. Therefore, careful interpretation of FA concerning diffusivity measures might be needed to evaluate disease-related WM changes.

5.2 Clinical Implications of FA in Brain White Matter

A study conducted by Zhan et al. in 2013 revealed that FA values depend on several factors to be clinically significant in medicine and suggested further imaging studies on white matter structures for assessing fibre orientation and its associated eigen- and FA values [20]. Another study on premature infants disclosed a powerful connection between FA values and age for fibres connected through the posterior end of the splenium of the CC [21]. The application of DTI and FA values has proven to be very helpful in identifying injuries to the corpus callus that indicate activity [22]. Significant variation was reported in a study where DTI analysis was done. FA values showed differences in males in contrast to females in the genu of the CC, whereas other diffusivity parameters did not show any variations [23]. A related study conducted on the correlation of ADC and FA values on the developing infant brain revealed that age plays an important role in the characterization between these two parameters [24]. A similar study on corpus callosum showed FA values on mid-sagittal DTI are higher compared to axial DTI values and FA values obtained from midsagittal DTI are more precise compared to axial DTI [25]. A research paper on the corpus callosum's adult ageing in the brain showed that FA values in older adults are lower than in younger adults [26]. The use of DTI in traumatic brain injury was used to detect vasogenic oedema in the genu more than in the corpus callosum splenium [27]. Different MRI field strengths (i.e. 1.5 and 3 T) show alteration in FA and ADC values, and values on 3 T show statistical significant values [28]. A study conducted on all normal seven segments of the CC in controls showed gender-independent FA heterogeneity, while patients suffering from multiple sclerosis showed decreased FA values [29]. FA maps and values were found to be very useful in detecting lacunar lesions in different regions of the corpus callosum [30]. Variations were seen in different ROI-based methods, and the circular ROI technique gave a better and higher repeatability rate compared to the freehand ROI [31]. A study on *b*-value and time of echo (TE) to determine the accuracy and repeatability of diffusion tensor-derived indices obtained at 1.5 T revealed that both of these factors influence results obtained in grey and white matter [32]. A study conducted on different 3 T magnets and higher angular resolution pulse sequences concluded that FA is the most comparable and reliable parameter than individual diffusivity parameters [33]. Another diffusion-tensor study found that FA levels in the superior longitudinal fasciculus of the left side decreased, which was essential in detecting depression abnormalities [34]. In a study conducted on FA and ADC values, the results showed regional variation in different areas of white matter [35]. The number of diffusion-weighted directions affects FA results; hence, this study suggested undertaking group and longitudinal studies utilizing the same DTI schemes with fixed directions [36]. A study conducted on developing an infant's brain concluded that FA and ADC values have a strong influence on the aged [24]. FA has been studied in relation to *b*-value, and it has been observed that a *b*-value of 1000 is the most reproducible in all areas of the brain, and FA values vary with different *b*-values [37]. A study conducted on the 3 T MR system on 20 regions of the brain showed that FA and ADC do not show a positive correlation between FA and age. It also states that field strength makes a slight difference in the measured FA values [8]. Functional DTI with task activation showed changes along white matter neural tracts of the brain [38]. A study conducted with a new DTI quantification model for fibre integrity showed FA values in the corticospinal tract with a high reproducibility [39]. The effects of SNR on diffusion tensor-derived FA values conclude that a minimum set threshold is a must for good and accurate DTI contrast at 1.5 T [40].

5.2.1 ROI Analysis for FA in the Brain

Some of the WM regions of the brain studied with DTI derivatives are listed below:

1. Tract-based spatial statistics method
2. Freehand ROI techniques
3. Fixed ROI techniques
4. Segmentation techniques
5. Voxel-based measurement and analysis

There are several motions and eddy current correction software used in advanced MRI scanners. The technique of a fixed and freehand ROI technique for investigating the brain white matter regions is most commonly used in [41]. The ROI-based technique is the most reliable technique for a clinical setting and diagnosis [42].

5.3 Quantitative Parameters Affecting FA Values

FA values are not measured in any specific units and range from 0 to 1. High FA values will be reflected by a greater degree of anisotropic motion. The number of diffusion weighing directions has an impact on FA values [43]. FA values are also affected by the *b*-values and echo time [37].

FA values are affected by both quantitative and qualitative parameters. Factors affecting FA values are the magnetic field strength, TR, TE, diffusion-weighted directions, coil type used, homogeneity of the magnet and so on. The main factors which quantitatively affect FA values are the *b*-value and TE. *b*—the value of 1000 is superior to other values and shows good reproducibility in most anatomic locations as shown by studies reported in literature [37].

FA decreases as *b*-value decreases, and FA increases as TE increase [32]. FA values are now used to observe, treat, and follow up on neurologically abnormal patients. FA values have been shown in clinical studies to be a reliable predictor of white matter abnormalities in ageing and neurological disorders [44].

5.4 Case Reports and Case Series Related to Diffusion-Tensor Imaging and Fractional Anisotropy Values

Studies conducted on *b*-value and time of echo (TE) to check for the accuracy and repeatability of diffusion tensor-derived indices obtained at 1.5 T revealed that both these factors affect results obtained in grey and white matter of the brain [32].

Hence, detailed published evidence using various combinations of *b*-value and TE will help inaccurate interpretation of FA values and design a fixed DTI protocol with *b*-value and TE combination to obtain consistent FA values.

5.4.1 Evidence on Influence of *b*-Value and TE on FA Values

5.4.1.1 *b*-Value Effects on FA

A study was conducted on 12 healthy volunteers which included (6M and 6F—mean age 38.4 ± 11.1 years) using two different *b*-values to check for age-related changes of FA, reproducibility and interrater agreement. The instrument used for imaging was a standard head coil for a 3-Tesla (T) Intera, Philips system. The DTI sequence used was spin-echo EPI, NEX = 2, TR = 5000 ms, TE = 90 ms, flip angle = 90°, slice thickness = 3 mm with zero gaps, FOV = 230 mm, acquisition matrix of 112 × 112 interpolated to 256 × 256, and diffusion-weighted directions used were 16 and *b*-values of 700 and 1000 s/mm^2, respectively. This study was performed after 2 weeks on the same subjects. FA measurements were done by two experienced neuroradiologists separately, using software provided by drawing ROIs. ROI placements were at the following locations—genu of the CC, splenium of the CC, right and left posterior internal capsule, left internal capsule and right thalamus along with right and left corticospinal tracts in the pons. The sizes of the ROIs used were 0.05 cm^2 (internal capsule and corticospinal tracts) and 0.20 cm^2 (corpus callosum and thalamus). There was no statistical difference found in both *b*-values except at the right internal capsule (mean FA = 0.702/0.728; *b* = 1000/700, *P* = 0.2) and anterior limb of the left internal capsule (mean FA = 0.617/0.745 and *b* = 1000/700, *P* = 0.5). No sex-related statistically relevant difference was found (*P* = 0.7). The significant age-related difference was only found at the genu of the CC (*P* = 0.04) and the left anterior limb of the internal capsule. Coming to an inter-rater agreement, only FA values (*P* = 0.001) in the splenium of the CC, right internal capsule and right thalamus showed very good agreement with a *b*-value of 1000 s/mm^2. Reproducibility in all anatomic regions was better with a *b*-value of 1000. Some important constraints of this study were (1) small sample size; (2) limited, i.e. only six, diffusion-weighted directions to determine FA values and (3) not checking the pathologic structures for any difference in reproducibility pattern [37].

5.4.1.2 *b*-Value and Time of Echo (TE) Effects on FA

In a similar study in 2012, *b*-value and TE were investigated for their effects on DTI-derived parameters, primarily AD, RD, MD, FA and principal eigenvector at 1.5 T MRI on both grey and white matter. This study was carried out on a 26-year-old male volunteer with no history of brain disease. The imaging system used was 1.5-Tesla (T) superconducting magnet with a six-channel phased-array head coil (Philips Medical Systems, Netherlands). The following imaging parameters were used with six *b*-values (250,500,750,1000,1500 and 2000 s/mm^2) and a fixed TE of 100 milliseconds (ms) for the first set and five TE values (80, 90, 100, 110 and 120 ms) and a fixed *b*-value of 750 s/mm^2 for the second set. A *b*-value of 750 s/mm^2 and TE 100 were taken separately for five datasets to get a reference. This experiment was carried out on the same subject three times in a row. On the obtained DTI indices, special automated software was used to correct the images from the motion artefact. Whole-brain coefficient of variation (CV) (MD) maps showed a decrease in MD with *b*-value but and increase with TE. The CV (MD) for white matter 12.2%

decreases with *b*-value 250 to 3.5% at *b*-value 2000. With a reduction in TE from 120 to 80 ms, CV (MD) in white matter decreased from 5.9% to 4.1%, respectively. According to the study's specific findings, Whole-brain FA decreases with *b*-values and marginally rises for *b*-values larger than 1000 s/mm^2, and prolonged TE leads to increased FA and lower SNR when utilizing voxel-wise analysis. The least CV (FA) was found in the white matter with a *b*-value of 1000, i.e. 11.5% compared to the *b*-value of 2000, i.e. 12.2%. The lowest CV (FA) for TE was found at 80 ms, i.e. 10.1%. Coming to the reproducibility of FA values, a *b*-value of 1000 and a reduced TE value were considered the best combination. According to the study, the accuracy and repeatability of DTI indices in both grey and white matter are affected by the *b*-value and TE [32].

5.4.1.3 High- and Low-Resolution DTI Effects on FA

In 2005, a study in Greece attempted to compare low- and high-resolution DTI sequences on FA and ADC measurements of normal brains. The main goal was to improve the SNR, acquisition time and spatial resolution of diffusion-tensor image sequences for routine clinical applications. The study included 20 healthy subjects with mean age of 18.6 years (range 17–19 years) who were scanned with a 1.5-Tesla full-body MRI unit (Sonata, Siemens Medical Solutions, Erlangen, Germany). A FLASH scout sequence was performed on all three planes, as well as a FLAIR axial turbo (TR/TE/TI/averages: 9000 ms/124 ms/2500 ms/2) and two axial tensor sequences. The first DTI sequence (DTI-A) was refined for time of acquisition, while the second sequence (DTI-B) was optimized for spatial resolution. Because the signal to noise ratio differed between the two sequences, FA and MD values differed significantly in the study. The study's limitations included overestimation of FA and MD values in similar imaging parameters [45].

5.4.1.4 An Animal Study on Time of Echo (TE) on FA

An animal study was carried out on rhesus monkeys (all males) to investigate the effects of echo time on brain WM diffusion quantification at 1.5 and 3 T MRI structures. The experiment was permitted by the institution's local animal care committee. The animals were given anaesthetic medications by intravenous injection. The imaging protocol used was a DTI sequence integrated with parallel acquisition techniques (iPAT). The other main parameters included were *b*-value = 1000 and six diffusion-weighted directions for image acquisition. These DTI sequences were repeated 12 times at 1.5 and 3 T with different TE ranging from 75 to 160 ms. T1-weighted images were also collected for anatomical correlation. The ROI technique was used to calculate the MD, FA, principal eigenvalues ($\lambda 1$) and transverse eigenvalues at the bilateral internal capsule. Statistical analysis was done using interclass correlation coefficients (ICC), Pearson's correlation coefficients and two-way repeated ANOVA. The study results revealed that FA and principal eigenvalues ($\lambda 1$) increased and transverse eigen ($\lambda 23$) values decreased with both TE at 1.5 and 3 T except for MD. ANOVA revealed that at 3 T, FA was significantly higher and MD and $\lambda 23$ were significantly lower than at 1.5 T. The study finally concluded that TE might influence the difference in diffusion quantification in brain white matter.

The study reported the following limitations: small sample size, use of animals, single study area for diffusion quantification and use of only six diffusion-weighted directions [46].

5.4.1.5 Animal Study (Rats)

In 2010, in China, studies explored the *b*-value dependency of DTI quantification and sensitivity in identifying brain tissue changes using rats. The data was gathered utilizing various *b*-values and 30 gradient directions on the rat brains at postnatal days 13, 21 and 120. Mean and directional diffusivities consistently decreased with the *b*-value in grey and white matter. FA levels changed minimally with *b*-value but also in a manner that was depending on age and tissue type, according to the study's findings. According to the Statistical analysis, FA sensitivity in identifying particular tissue changes was impacted by *b*-values. As a result, the choice of *b*-value influences FA values, and caution must be exercised when interpreting DTI indices in clinical patients [47].

5.4.1.6 The Influence of SNR on FA

In the United States, Jonathan et al. in 2007 studied the impact of SNR on the accuracy and reproducibility of FA, MD and primary eigenvector measurements at 1.5 T. Only one 24-year-old healthy volunteer was included in the study. For image acquisition, a Philips 1.5-T Intera system with an eight-channel phased-array head coil was used. The DTI protocol used a multislice, single-shot EPI sequence with a 90-degree flip angle, TR/TE = 3632 ms/100 ms, *b*-value = 1000 and 30 diffusion-weighted directions. MATLAB was used to process DTI datasets. The study's findings revealed that FA increased as SNR decreased. Overall, obtaining accurate and exact FA values in grey matter needs a greater SNR than quantification of FA values in white matter. As a result, SNR of DTI sequences, in general, should be considered when using FA values in clinical patients. The study's limitations included single sample size and a lack of comparison in multicentric studies. The authors advocated for larger sample size longitudinal comparison studies as well as the development of a standard protocol for acquiring DTI images [40].

5.4.1.7 DTI Parameter Effects of *b*-Value and Field Strength

In 2012, a study was carried out in the United Kingdom to investigate the relationship between *b*-value and field strength on diffusion-tensor parameters on eight healthy subjects who were scanned using 1.5- and 3-T MRI units. The major purpose of the study was to determine how SNR and field strength affected FA values. Data were collected at 1.5 and 3 T, with *b*-values of 0, 1000, 2000 and 3000 in each of the 20 diffusion-weighted directions. FA values were computed using various *b*-value sets. The genu and splenium of CC, the bilateral CS, the putamen and the thalamus, among other white and grey matter areas of the brain, were examined for field strength and *b*-value effects. The study found that as the *b*-value in white matter increased, FA decreased. Furthermore, in extremely dense white matter brain areas, univariate analysis indicated a substantial increase in FA along with increasing field strength. The study results indicate variation in diffusion parameters at 1.5 and 3 T, and a *b*-value of 1000 is recommended for consistent and reliable FA values [48].

5.5 FA in Normative Healthy Brain White Matter

Limited studies are reported in the literature on normative FA among different regions of the brain grey and white matter. The effects of TE, *b*-value, SNR and diffusion-weighted directions on FA values have also been reported in studies. A detailed correlation of FA values with different age groups also remains unexplored. Thus, a shred of detailed evidence on normative values of FA of the different regions of the normal brain will be very useful clinically for neurosurgeons, neurologists and oncologists in pre- and post-operative management.

The incidence of complex brain diseases is increasing at an alarming rate worldwide. Advanced MR imaging techniques must be utilized as a routine imaging protocol to detect these diseases. Limited and unexplored studies in DTI have encouraged in-depth research work on FA values. There is still a gap in the literature, and a standardized set of FA values in normal brain tissues and grey and white matter were missing. FA values of any diseased areas are considered abnormal only when compared to contralateral corresponding brain FA values. Hence when there is diffuse brain involvement, we need to compare with a normative reference standard FA range. Clinical studies reported have recommended FA values for detection of neurological abnormalities [26, 44]. These studies reported showed positivity in using FA values for early detection and diagnosis in the brain white and grey matter, and hence obtaining a normative database on FA values will be very useful. Detailed data on normative FA values in different age groups will be explained in-depth in the current and upcoming chapters on diffusion-tensor imaging and normative FA.

5.5.1 Evidence of Human Studies on Normative and Neurodegenerative Disorders

5.5.1.1 Application of DTI and FA

The subsection of this chapter deals with evidence on some key findings on normative FA in different regions of the brain grey and white matter. It also throws light on the clinical importance of FA in neurology, neurosurgery and other specialities.

5.5.1.2 Normal Pressure Hydrocephalus and DTI (FA)

Szczepek et al. [49] studied normal pressure hydrocephalus and brain atrophy. To distinguish between normal pressure hydrocephalus and brain atrophy, the DTI method was utilized. Patients with idiopathic normal pressure hydrocephalus, cerebral atrophy and healthy controls were included in this investigation. To obtain diffusion-tensor images, this study used 1.5- and 3-T MRI scanners. FA values were calculated using a tract spatial statistics region of interest technique based on computed tract-based spatial statistics. The following brain areas were evaluated: fibre commissural lateral ventricles, corpus callosum minor forceps, cingulum, optic radiation and corpus callosum minor forceps. The main findings were that, when compared to the cerebral atrophy and control groups, FA values in the hydrocephalus group differed significantly in the posterior cingulate and forceps minor of the corpus callosum. The study's main finding was that white matter tract changes in specific regions of the brain distinguish it from cerebral atrophy and control brains [49].

5.5.1.3 Normative FA Using Small and High-Resolution Diffusion-Tensor Images

Papanikolaou et al. [45] compared sequences of 20 people with 18.5 years as the mean age (range 17–20 years) with small and high-resolution diffusion-tensor images to determine FA and MD readings on the ordinary human brain. The main goal of this study was to develop DTI sequences for routine clinical situations in terms of SNR, spatial resolution and time. A 1.5-T (Siemens Sonata Germany) whole-body MRI scanner was used for imaging with a maximum gradient strength of 40 mT/m and a slew rate of 200 T m^{-1} S^{-1}. For image acquisition, a quadrature head coil was used. For image acquisition, two DTI protocols were used. The first DTI-A was used for a time, while the second DTI-B was used for spatial resolution, and the entire brain was analysed. Both protocols used a *b*-value of 1000, TEs of 85 and 94 and diffusion-weighted directions of 6. A dedicated workstation and software were used for image pre- and post-processing (MEDx, SPM 99 MODEL Medical Numerics, Va, USA). This study found that both DTI sequences clearly defined white matter structures. The DTI-A protocol was used to calculate higher ADC values and vice versa. DTI-A protocol was used to demonstrate lower FA-based areas and vice versa. When compared to relative anisotropy and volume ratio, FA is regarded as a superior and more robust quantification technique [45]. Significant differences in ADC and FA were discovered in this study. "Increased image noise may be one of the primary causes of FA and ADC quantification errors" [50]. "The DTI-B protocol had a lower SNR than the DTI-A protocol, resulting in an overvaluation of FA in white matter and an underestimating of ADC" [45].

5.5.1.4 FA and White Matter Alteration in Idiopathic Standard Hydrocephalus Pressure (INPH)

Koyama et al. [51] used a voxel-based fractional anisotropy (FA) method to detect changes in white matter caused by idiopathic standard hydrocephalus pressure (INPH). INPH patients and controls were included in the study, with a total of ten subjects in each group (>60 years old). Gait disturbance, dementia and urinary incontinence were all diagnosed in INPH patients. MRI, chest radiography, electrocardiography and blood samples were all part of the study's routine protocol. The MR scanner used was a 3-T Siemens Erlangen with a 32-channel head coil, and the typical DTI sequence used a *b*-value of 1000 and a time interval of 83 ms. For diagnostic purposes, T2-weighted spin echo and T1-weighted images were also obtained. Image preprocessing included removing motion artefacts, and FA values were generated in the forceps minor (anterior portion of the corpus callosum), white matter tracts and bilateral corticospinal tracts using specialized software. The ROI techniques were used to compute FA values. The authors reported that FA in the forceps minor was lower in INPH patients (0.504) than in the control group (0.632), but no significant differences were found in the corticospinal tract. Within ROIs, conventional *t*-tests were used to compare the two groups, and the Spearman's rank correlation test was used to determine the relationship between clinical symptoms and FA values in INPH patients. A *p*-value less than 0.05 was considered statistically significant. The study had some limitations, including (a) a very small sample size and (b) the inclusion of patients with no history of Parkinson's or Alzheimer's disease, and further research in this area was suggested [51].

5.5.1.5 Radiofrequency Coils and FA

Giannelli et al. (2010) used two different radiofrequency head coils to compare MD and FA values at 1.5 T. The author used 14 people who have never had a neurological condition before (seven males and seven females with mean age of 31 years, age range 24–42 years), and each subject was scanned twice with two different head coils. A 1.5-T Signa Hdxt MR system with a maximum gradient strength of 50 mT/m and a slew rate of 150 T/m/s was used for imaging. The imaging DTI sequence was a spin EPI sequence with $b = 1000$ s/mm^2 and TE = 84 ms and 31 diffusion-weighted directions. For imaging, a quadrature head coil from a birdcage (Coil-A) and an eight-channel head coil array (Coil-B) were employed. The FA and MD values of grey and white matter structures in the corpus callosum splenium (CCS), inner capsule (IC), middle cerebral peduncle (MCP), globus pallidus (GP), thalamus (TH), caudate (CA) and putamen (PU) were determined. The FA and MD values were calculated using the linear and non-linear least squares techniques. The Wilcoxon test for paired samples, with and without Bonferroni adjustments, was used to assess variations in DTI measurements. The authors observed a 30% increase in overall SNR in Coil-B when compared to Coil-A. When the other values in Coil-B were compared to the other values in Coil-A, the mean FA (SCC, IC and TH), mean MD (IC, CP, GP and TH), FA standard deviation (CP, MCP, GP and CA) and MD standard deviation (IC, CP, TH and PV) results decreased *p* (correlated) 0.05 and *p* (uncorrelated) <0.05 in several grey and white matter regions of the human brain. According to the study, in comparison with the quadrature birdcage head coil, the eight-channel head coil delivered specific and reliable measurements of DTI-derived indices [52].

5.5.1.6 Normative FA in an Adult Healthy Population

Sexton et al. [16] investigated changes in white matter structures during ageing using DTI. A total of 203 healthy adults between the ages of 20 and 84 were studied using DTI imaging and tract-based spatial statistics to determine changes in FA values in brain white matter compared to AD, RD and MD as an individual's age increased. Other studies comparing the ages of healthy participants and at-risk populations were suggested by the study [16].

Brander et al. [35] used DTI of the healthy brain to investigate normative FA and ADC values at 1.5 and 3 T. The primary goal of the study was to determine normal FA and ADC values in adults, as well as the intra and inter-observer reproducibility of the measurements. Forty volunteers, 26 of whom were women and 14 of whom were men (mean age 38.3, SD 11.6 years), underwent brain MRI and DTI scans, 30 of whom were scanned with 3-T scanners and 10 with 1.5-T scanners. Three-Tesla Siemens trio and 1.5-T Siemens Avanto MRI scanners were used. A head coil with two channels was used. T1-weighted 3D inversion recovery (IR); axial T2 turbo spin echo; and FLAIR axial, AxT2*, T2 axial and axial SWI were acquired as routine MRI sequences. DTI protocols included a single short diffusion-weighted echo-planar imaging sequence with 3-T parameters of TE = 92 ms, $b = 0$ and 1000 s/mm^2 and 20 diffusion gradient orientations, as well as 1.5-T parameters of TE = 96 ms, $b = 0$ and 1000 s/mm^2 and 12 diffusion gradient orientations. Two observers (a physicist and a neuroradiologist) used circular ROIs to calculate FA and ADC values on the following anatomic regions: basal pons, mesencephalon, cerebral peduncle, the posterior rim of the internal capsule, corona radiata, centrum semiovale, and corpus callosum (genu, corpus and splenium). Both observers repeated the ROI measurements in ten subjects at 3 T. For calculating FA and ADC, the mean and standard deviation were calculated using the following statistical analysis: The *t*-test for equality of means was employed to analyse gender differences, and the paired *t*-test was used to analyse interhemispheric differences. To assess inter- and intraobserver agreement, the Bland-Altman test was used. Mean FA ranged from 0.52 (right corona radiata) to 0.87 (corpus callosum and splenium) for 1.5 T and 0.48–0.86 for 3 T. ADC ranged from 0.64×10^{-3} to 0.86×10^{-3} mm^2/s for 1.5 T and 0.65×10^{-3} mm^2/s (left corona radiata) to 0.85×10^{-3} mm^2/s for 3 T (corpus callosum body). There were no gender differences in FA values discovered. There were no differences in the region mean between 3 T (30 subjects) and 1.5 T (10 subjects) in the analysis of the results. Only FA values in the corona radiata and ADC in the capsule showed statistically significant differences in interhemispheric differences. Results for best inter-observer variation of 40 subjects for FA were taken in the genu and splenium of the corpus callosum (CV% 5.2 vs. 6.5) and lowest in the centrum semiovale (CV% right 28.4, left 25.1) and for ADC least in right corona radiata (CV% 8.1) and splenium of corpus callosum (CV% 8.8%) and lowest in the right mesencephalon (CV% 17.9). FA had the highest reproducibility for intraobserver variation in the genu and splenium of the CC, while ADC had the same in the genu, splenium and right internal capsule. Regional variation in FA values is known to exist in the brain parenchyma, and FA values are usually higher in the CC due to the dense network of white matter fibres [8, 53]. In most published articles, FA values for white matter are in the range of 0.5–0.8 and ADC 0.7–0.9 × 10^{-3} mm^2/s [9–11, 37, 54]. The small sample size was the limitation of this study [35].

Lee et al. (2008) conducted a study to determine normative FA and ADC in healthy volunteers in 20 different regions of the brain. Previous studies conducted normative FA and ADC at 3 T [28, 55] with a limited anatomical region and with a limited sample size. The study included 31 volunteers (mean age 36 years) ranging in age from 19 to 62 (15 males and 15 females), 5 of whom were scanned twice within 90 days to check for repeatability. A 3-T Philips Intera MR system with a maximum amplitude of 40 mT/m and a rise time of 20 milliseconds (ms) was used. To acquire data, only a six-channel head coil was used. A single-shot spin echo, the echo-planar sequence with 32 non-collinear directions (max *b* factor = 1000 s/mm^2, TE = 86 ms), was used in the DTI sequence, which was repeated three times. In addition to this routine MR sequence, a 3D rapid gradient magnetization prepared Sagittal FLAIR and T2-weighted sequence was acquired. In order to correct motion and eddy currents, pride tool of Philips was used. The ROI was drawn in all the following regions of the brain: the medulla pyramid, the middle cerebellar peduncle, the superior cerebellar peduncle, the forceps minor, the anterior limb of the internal capsule, the genu and splenium of the corpus callosum globus, the pallidus, the anterior thalamus, the posterior thalamus and the corona radiate. The study's age groups ranged from 19 to 39 years.

FA and ADC were compared right and left using paired *t*-tests, and to look for any age correlation, Pearson's correlation test was used. A one-way variance analysis was performed to look for gender differences in FA and ADC. A paired *t*-test was used to check for repeatability in five contributors." At 25 °C, the mean ADC of distilled water was $2.21 \pm 0.02 \times 10^{-3}$ mm^2/s, which is consistent with Jansen et al. $2.20 \pm 0.04 \times 10^{-3}$ mm^2/s" [56]. The maximum FA was found in the corpus callosum, which was followed by a cerebral peduncle, posterior limb of the internal capsule and middle cerebellar peduncle, with the deep nuclei having the lowest FA. ADC values were generally low except for fornix, optic radiation and tract. To summarize, neither FA nor ADC (gender or age difference) showed any statistically significant difference, and normative data of FA and ADC in 20 different regions of the brain were presented, which will aid in the diagnosis of various neurologic conditions.

5.5.1.7 FA and Brain Myelination in Healthy Volunteers

Löbel et al. [57] carried out a long-term study to determine normative values of ADC, RA, FA and eigenvalues in various brain regions to better understand the process of myelination in healthy patients. Patients in the age group of 3 weeks to 19 years were included, and exclusion criteria involved patients that may have possible white matter abnormalities. A 1.5-T MR Magnetom Siemens scanner with transmit-receive head coil was used for imaging. DTI TRSE-EPI-DTI sequence with $b = 0$ and 1000 s/mm^2 and TE of 100 ms was used. Data pre-analysis was done using MATLAB (The Maths works, Natick, MA, USA) to find region values and calculate other diffusion parameters. ROIs were placed in 12 various parts of the brain in both hemispheres, and the lateral ventricle was taken as a reference measurement. The genu and splenium of the CC, anterior and posterior limbs, internal capsule, anterior and posterior pons and WM regions (frontal, temporal, parietal and occipital WM) were all assessed. The Spearman' correlation coefficient and regression analysis were used for statistical analysis. Mean ROI sizes varied from 17 to 45 interpolated voxels. Findings included mean values ranging from 71.6×10^{-5}

(posterior pons) to 90.3 × 10^{-5} mm^2/s (parietal white matter) for ADC and 0.32 (inferior frontal white matter) to 0.94 (splenium of corpus callosum) for RA and varied between 0.36 (inferior frontal white matter) and 0.81 (splenium of corpus callosum) for FA. Mean values with lateral ventricles measured 303.2 × 10^{-5} mm^2/s, 0.21 and 0.25 for ADC (average), RA and FA, respectively. There was a strong influence of age in anterior regions (genu of the corpus callosum, anterior pons, anterior portion of the internal capsule, frontal white matter) as compared to regions lying in the posterior region (temporal and occipital white matter) and also superiorly (superior frontal and parietal white matter). The study concluded that ADC (average), FA and eigenvalues decreased whereas RA increased with age. Also within a region, different diffusion parameters showed the different amounts of changes. Age differed in both anisotropy indices (RA and FA). Limitations of the study included recruiting patients in the study, and secondly, this was a retrospective study, so it could not characterize individual varieties. Based on the patient's age, the ROI size varied within the same patient in FA values. Age-related differences in this study were very less and will not have a great effect in detecting the course of myelination. Thirdly, the direction of the diffusion tensor was not considered. Further studies should consider evaluation of both FA and RA together or correct for degree of anisotropy. The study concluded that the myelination process is a challenge as ADC, RA and FA act differently for microstructural changes [57].

In the United States, a DTI study of healthy ageing was linked to access age-related differences in multiple measures of white matter integrity in 2010. Multiple diffusivity measures, namely FA, AD and RD, were compared between young and healthy older adults in this study to determine how age affects white matter in the brain. The 3.0-Tesla MRI system was used to scan the participants (Siemens Magnetom Trio, Erlangen, Germany). Then, in 35 orthogonal directions, two 35-direction diffusion-weighted echo-planar imaging sequences were acquired using gradient values of $b = 0$ and $b = 1000$ s/mm^2. The study showed two patterns (radial increase only and radial/axial increase) as well as one distinct pattern (radial increase/axial decrease). Furthermore, the anterior-posterior gradient of age differences in white matter integrity was consistent with larger age differences in FA in frontal white matter. Some of the limitations mentioned are the lack of tractography and the use of the TBSS method for calculating FA values [58].

Kochunov et al. [59] compared the relationship between FA of white matter and other cerebral health indices in normal ageing in San Antonia, USA. The authors hypothesized that the decline in white matter health could be linked to changes in a number of other indicators. A total of 31 healthy ageing subjects (12 men and 19 women) ranging in age from 57 to 82 years were studied for the relationship between hemispheric whole-brain, FA corpus callosum and grey matter (GM) density, sulcal span and T2-hyperintense white matter quantity. FA values were computed using the DTI dataset and tract-based spatial statistics. Age controlled correlation analysis was used for statistical analysis. Whole-brain FA values correlated significantly with the subject's average grey matter thickness and negatively with hyperintense white matter volume. The left FA and left grey matter thickness had a significant intra-hemispheric correlation ($r = 0.6$, $P \leq 0.01$). The study concluded that late demyelinating brain regions are associated with age-related degenerative changes [59].

A similar study on age and gender on white matter integrity was conducted in Tokyo in 2011 with a large sample to investigate age-related changes, gender differences and age-by-sex relationships in white matter integrity (FA, AD, and RD) across the brain. This study included 857 healthy subjects (average age = 56.1 ± 9.9 years; age range = 24.9–84.8 years). At 3 T, all subjects were scanned. The TBSS method was used to investigate the effects of age and gender on FA, AD and RD in the white matter. The findings revealed that FA correlated negatively with age, whereas AD and RD correlated positively with age. There were no gender differences in the white matter's ageing process [60].

In the year 2010, a longitudinal study using the TBSS technique was conducted in London to investigate the structural decline in white matter in normal ageing. The study included a total of 106 adults, who were healthy (55 males and 51 females; age range: 50–90; average age: 69 years). A total of 84 participants (48 men and 36 women; ages 55–91 years; mean age = 71 years). DWI images were acquired on the 1.5-T General Electric Signa MRI using a diffusion-sensitized spin-echo EPI series. To study local age-related structural changes, longitudinal variations in FA, AD and RD were investigated utilizing standard space 1D coronal slice profiles and 2D column maps, as well as 3D TBSS on a voxel-by-voxel basis at baseline and 2-year follow-up. The CC (genu, body, splenium), cingulum (anterior part, posterior section), internal capsule (anterior limb, posterior limb), external capsule and superior corona radiata were all studied using the ROI approach. With age as the dependent variable, statistical analysis was conducted employing linear and quadratic correlation patterns. A paired *t*-test approach was used to assess the longitudinal change between baseline and follow-up. The difference between baseline and follow-up was analysed using linear regression, using age at baseline as the dependent variable. To see if the longitudinal change increased with age, linear regression was used on the difference between baseline and follow-up, with age at baseline as a dependent variable. Each risk factor (BMI, diastolic blood pressure, systolic blood pressure, cholesterol level, years of smoking pack and volume of WMH) was investigated in the same way, with the difference between baseline and monitoring serving as the independent variable in linear regression and each risk factor (BMI, diastolic blood pressure, systolic blood pressure, cholesterol level, years of smoking pack and volume of WMH) serving as the dependent variable. DTI can identify age-related changes in WM structure in a short period of time, according to the findings, and longitudinal analyses demonstrate significant changes in white matter integrity across the brain over 2 years, with no indication of a faster deterioration in frontal lobe areas. Along with the use of TBSS procedures, one of the study's shortcomings was the use of AD and RD [61].

In 2009, a Tokyo-based study developed a database of conventional diffusion-tensor metrics of cerebral WM fibres such as the uncinate fasciculus (UF), posterior cingulum (PC), fornix and corticospinal tract (CST) for healthy teenagers using tract-specific DTI analysis. It included 100 healthy people and measured MD and FA values. The age associations were evaluated using Pearson's correlation analysis. To compare hemispheric asymmetry, paired *t*-testing was used. The study found a substantial positive relationship between age and MD in the right UF and bilateral fornices, as well as an adverse relationship between ages with FA in the bilateral fornices. FA of UF (right > left) and MD of CST (left > right) showed hemispheric asymmetry. As a result, the study provided a normative chart of FA and MD values [62].

5.5.1.8 Normative FA of Brain Structures in Children/Infants

Snook et al. [12] conducted a study on children to determine their neurodevelopment using DTI. MD and FA values were assessed in 13 different brain structures across 30 different brain regions. The study used 2 healthy groups of volunteers: 32 children aged 8–12 years (18 females and 14 males) and 28 young adults (aged 21–27 years) with no psychiatric disease or neurological injury. For image acquisition, a 1.5-T Siemens Sonata system with dual spin echo, SS-EPI and TE = 86 ms and *b*-value = 1000 was used. ADC and FA values were collected from the following brain areas, which were further classified into four tissue types: (1) CC's genu and splenium, lower limb of the internal capsule, anterior limb of the internal capsule corona radiate, external capsule and centrum semiovale which are all examples of major white matter; (2) subcortical white matter in gyri: a sample of five gyri including the right superior frontal gyrus, right supramarginal gyrus, right middle occipital gyrus, left superior temporal gyrus and left postcentral gyrus; (3) cortical grey matter: a thin band around the subcortical white matter gyri; and (4) deep grey matter: part of the brain, globes pallidus, putamen and head of the caudate nucleus. Image analysis was carried out with the help of MR vision and the Winchester software. The paired *t*-test was utilized to compare left and right asymmetry differences, and a correlation analysis was done for both FA and ADC vs. age in children (8–12 years) and young adults (21–27 years). In a group analysis, the performance of each brain area across the groups of children and young adults was compared. In both ADC and FA values, there was just a little hemispheric asymmetry. Correlation analysis revealed an increase in FA in the genu, splenium, corona radiate, putamen and caudate nucleus head. In children, there was no evident decrease in FA with age, while ADC showed decreased values in 9 out of 13 regions, whereas there was a minimal change in the age range of 21–27 years in young adults, with an increase in ADC in the right globus pallidus and an increase in FA in the right centrum semiovale. FA values increased in 11 of 13 structures from children to young adults, with a decrease in FA in the right centrum semiovale. In 12 of the 13 structures, ADC showed a decrease in value. To summarize, FA rises in 5 of the 13 structures tested from 8 years to young adulthood, while ADC decreases in 9 of the 13 structures studied [12].

In the year 2003, in healthy neonates and adults, a comparative study on regional white matter diffusion was done in the northern state of Carolina in the United States using a 3-T head only MR unit. The main goal of the study was to look for age-related and regional differences in FA and ADC in normal adult and neonatal brains. A single-shot diffusion-tensor sequence was used to enrol 8 healthy adults and 20 healthy neonates in the study. White matter (WM) tract ADC and FA maps were obtained. The ROI technique was used in both grey and white matter brain regions. The student *t*-test was used as the statistical test for comparing FA and ADC in both groups. The Tukey multiple-comparison test was used to assess FA and ADC in various brain areas in the adult and newborn groups. There were statistically significant differences in both grey and white matter, with an increase in ADC and a decrease in FA. The study concluded that in neonates, there were regional disparities in FA and ADC levels that were not seen in adults [63].

In 2011, a DTI study of white matter maturation in childhood and adolescence was undertaken in South Korea. The goal of this study was to test two hypotheses: The first was that FA and ADC values vary during infancy and adolescence, and the second was that less mature white matter (WM) regions change quicker than more mature WM regions. A total of 87 healthy children (50 girls and 37 boys; mean age, 11.2 ± 3.6 years; range, 4.2–17.7 years) were subjected to a six-direction DTI sequence at a 3-T unit. Overall, during childhood and adolescence, FA values continue to climb while ADC values diminish [64].

5.5.1.9 Magnetic Field Strengths and FA

Huisman et al. [28] performed a study to investigate the effect of magnetic field strengths on DTI metrics, FA and ADC, as well as whether magnetic field-related variations in brain tissue T2 relaxation times affect DTI measurements. Twelve healthy volunteers (10 men, 2 women; age range, 26–31 years) without a history of neurological or systemic disease were subjected to a 1.5-T scan (Magnetom Siemens) and 3-T (Magnetom Trio) MRI scanners within 2 h using a standardized polarized head coil. The 3D T1-weighted MPRAGE sequence was acquired before the DTI sequence. The DTI sequence used was a DW single-shot spin-echo EPI sequence with $b = 0$ and $b = 1000$ and TE = 91 and 125 ms, respectively. MATLAB 6.5 was used for image processing. Freehand ROIs were put in the following anatomical areas of the brain by an experienced neuroradiologist: genuine inner capsule, posterior capsule limb, centrum semiovale, thalamus, caudate nucleus head, splenium and corpus callus truncus. The fine bilateral measurements for each location except the corpus callosum were averaged. SNR measurements were made on both field strengths and the standard deviation of noise in the backdrop areas outside the head, which were devoid of artefacts, using a 5 × 5 pixel ROI positioned at the thalamus. To compare data, the paired "*t*-test" was utilized. Using two different TEs of 1.5 and 3 T, there were no statistically relevant variations in FA and ADC. When compared to 3 T, SNR at 1.5 T was 19.1% higher. When 1.5-T and 3-T ADC values were compared, there was a statistically significant decrease in both grey and white matter. However, FA values in both grey and white matter increased statistically significantly. FA is one of the noise-resistant and robust scalars of the diffusion anisotropy [3, 7]. Some noted limitations of this study included a small sample size and comparing FA and ADC with normative values obtained from the same field strengths. The study concluded that at higher field strengths from 1.5 to 3 T, lower ADC and higher FA values were obtained [28].

5.5.1.10 MR Magnets and FA as a Robust Diffusivity Measure

Fox et al. [33] conducted a study using different MR magnets to find the reliability of FA and MD values. Two volunteers (both men, 35 years) were imaged using five 3-T MR magnets in different locations: three trios (Siemens) and two signals (GE). In addition, one person was imaged twice during the course of 2 years (using one of the Siemens 3 T). Imaging protocol used was T1 MPRAGE and twice refocused spin-echo DTI with TE = 100 ms and $b = 0$ s/mm^2 and $b = 1000$ s/mm^2 with 33 non-linear diffusion-weighted directions. Image registration was done using iterated closest point algorithm. For both the subjects, 16 ROIs were drawn on areas of the corpus callosum (genu and splenium), periventricular white matter (parietal and occipital), deep white matter (frontal, parietal and occipital), cortical grey matter (posterior parietal and occipital) and deep grey matter (putamen). ROI size varied from 182 to 742 mm^3. The highest concordance and reliability were found for FA (0.96) followed by longitudinal and parallel diffusivity and the weakest for ADC. Study observations state that FA is the best followed by component diffusivities as a higher priority outcome than regional ADC. Apart from this, a high field magnet and 33 non-linear directions were used to provide a robust diffusion estimate [65]. "Some previous studies used higher and lower diffusion directions, 3–6% CV in FA and MD using 60 directions at 1.5 T and 1.9% CV for FA in corpus callosum using 6 directions at 1.5 T" [66, 67]. The short sample size and various ROI sizes used for FA value estimate were some of the study's drawbacks.

5.5.1.11 FA and MD Using SNR Measurements

Hunsche et al. [55] used SNR measurements to determine the differences in FA and ADC at 1.5 and 3 T. The study included seven healthy volunteers (three males and four females aged 32 years' ± 2SD in the range of 30–36 years) with no previous history of neurological disease. For the phantom study, a spherical water phantom with a diameter of 18 cm doped with copper sulphate was used. Image acquisition was carried out using a 1.5-T and 3-T GE Echospeed MRI unit. A diffusion-weighted single-shot spin echo-planar sequence was used for DTI imaging, with TE = 90 ms and *b*-value = 0 and 900 in healthy volunteers and $b = 500$ in phantom imaging. DTI image processing was done on a separate workstation (Sun Ultra spark 60; sun microsystem) using software created at Stanford University's Lucas MRS Centre. To compare FA and ADC values at increasing SNR, the computations were performed four times with an increasing number of averaged repeats in the human investigation. Using ROI analysis in data analysis, the influence of field strength and SNR on FA and ADC was studied. FA and ADC statistical significance at 1.5 and 3 T were calculated using paired *t*-tests for each ROI. SNR was greater than 1.5 T in a human study at 3 T. To summarize diffusion-tensor MR, FA is higher in white matter than in grey matter. When compared to 1.5-T imaging, 3-T imaging gives improved picture resolution and a shorter imaging duration due to a 40% increase in SNR. At 1.5 and 3 T, there was no discernible difference between FA and ADC [55].

5.5.1.12 Diffusion-Weighted Directions and FA

Giannelli et al. [43] studied the diffusion-weighted direction numbers effects on FA and MD brain DTI maps in Italy. The study's primary goal was to look at the relationship between diffusion-weighted directions and anatomical structure accuracy and contrast. In high and low anisotropy segmented brain areas, FA and MD mean values were assessed. Furthermore, the CNR variance ratio between white matter and nearby regions was estimated. The experiment was carried out with a 1.5-T GE system, a gradient strength of 40 mT/m and a slew rate of 150 T/m/s. A standard quadrature head coil with a 26-cm diameter was employed for image acquisition. For image acquisition, a DWI-SE-EPI sequence was used. To reduce inter-subject bias, the study included six healthy volunteers, with an equal number of males and females of comparable age (29 ± 4) who had no previous neurological disease. The following was the imaging protocol that was used: The DWI-SE-EPI sequence had a TR of 8000 ms, a TE of 79 ms, a *b*-value of 1000 s/mm^2 and a total of 55 diffusion-weighted directions. The scan covered the area between the cervical bulbar junction and the centrum semiovale. SNR and CNR were measured in each anatomical region for each DTI dataset. To post-process the FA and MD maps, MATLAB version 6.5 was used. The non-parametric Friedman's test was used to analyse statistical data using one-way repeated measures analysis of variation (ANOVA). The relationship between FA and MD data values and the number of diffusion-weighted directions was investigated using Pearson' (P) and Spearman's (S) rank correlation tests. SNR decreases as N (DW direction number) increases and vice versa. To summarize, when DTI acquisition schemes with varied diffusion-weighted directions were applied, the study discovered that MD human brain values did not differ significantly, whereas FA values did. The number of diffusion-weighted directions increased the FA of high anisotropic structures, such as white matter, but the number of diffusion-weighted directions lowered the FA of low anisotropic areas. Similarly, the contrast to signal difference ratio among main white matter and the nearby regions increased significantly as the number of diffusion-weighted directions increased. The authors suggested that longitudinal and group comparison studies be conducted on all subjects using the same DTI scheme with a fixed number of diffusion-weighted directions. One of the study's limitations was the use of a single MRI system [43].

5.5.1.13 Q-Ball Imaging and FA

Various qualitative and quantitative factors influence different DTI imaging indices, such as FA and ADC. Caiazzo et al. (2015) conducted a comparison of high and low angular resolution diffusion-weighted MRI protocols for the investigation of brain white matter in Berlin using various Q-ball imaging models. Q-ball is a common information model used to quantify white matter anisotropy in diffusion-weighted MRI research. The goal of this model was to investigate human brain DW-MRI images from different protocols in 12 different brain white matter areas using single or double fibre models for white matter voxels. The study included seven healthy volunteers (two females and five males; mean age 27, 28 ± 5.38) who were scanned with a 3-T GE SIGNA HDXT MR magnet with an eight-channel head coil. All participants provided ethical clearance and informed consent. Imaging protocol for whole-brain DTI was done using a GRE echo EPI low number of diffusion direction, TR =10,000 ms, TE = 83.2 ms and *b*-value = 1000 s/mm^2 with 32 directions and high number of diffusion directions with TR = 16,000 ms, TE = 104 ms and *b*-value = 3000 s/mm^2 with 52 diffusion-weighted directions. MATLAB software was used for data analysis and image processing. The volume of interest analysis was done in advanced FMRIB FSL software. The white matter region studied were as follows: corpus callosum, corticospinal tract, superior and inferior longitudinal fissure, uncinate fasciculus, cingulum and fornix. The study reported that the anisotropy FA and fibre length and density produced higher values for higher angular weighted imaging compared to lower angular weighted imaging. The mean difference in echo time in both protocols did not show any impact on the image quality. *b*-Value provided the most consistent fibre orientation estimation in the presence of noise. Higher angular resolution weighting imaging had a limitation of longer acquisition time compared to its predecessor. The other limitation reported was a very small sample size [68].

5.5.1.14 Decreasing FA with an Increase in Age

In the year 2006, a narrative review on brain white matter and ageing was conducted in the United States to investigate the following hypotheses: (1) the anteroposterior gradient, (2) bilateral recruitment of brain systems via the corpus callosum for frontally based task execution and (3) front cerebellar synergism. The study's main purpose was to find age-related declines in FA in white matter in normal healthy people. The drop was shown to be equal in men and women, linear from approximately the age of 20, and has frontal distribution. Future directions include the use of DTI tractography and functional imaging to help dissect the brain regions that are active during task performance. The study could not reach a definitive conclusion about the relationship between the ageing brain and the factors that influence it, but it did report some important findings. The deterioration of brain integrity with age is most noticeable in the prefrontal regions. To maintain youthful performance levels, elderly persons may utilize brain areas that the young do not use, which are generally bilaterally distributed. Given the extensive circuitry of frontal systems, the cerebellum may provide additional compensation for age-related declines in executive or attentional functions. As a result, age-related degeneration of white matter systems might be a possible mechanism for age-related functional decline. White matter mediated neural system hypotheses of ageing brain structure and function emerged from recent DTI findings and conceptualizations of neural causes of cognitive decline in ageing: (1) the anteroposterior gradient of ageing, (2) bilateral recruitment of brain systems via the corpus callosum for frontally based task execution and (3) frontocerebellar synergism. These hypotheses are not completely exclusive, but they do provide a platform for testing questions concerning brain systems that are recruited when those employed in youth are changed by ageing. The consequences of normal adult ageing, unlike those of neurodegenerative disorders and neurological events, are mild, build up slowly and can be difficult to detect with typical structural neuroimaging techniques. In vivo identification of patterns of sparing and compromise of white matter integrity in normal ageing, which is subtle on the macrostructural level but more reliably observable on the microstructural level, is supported by a growing corpus of DTI research. DTI, as a measure of brain tissue quality, enables the analysis of regional patterns of neural circuitry degeneration associated with ageing that is not possible with other imaging techniques. Quantitative tractography has the potential to be especially useful for delineating and assessing neural circuitry integrity and functional correlates. Future research that combines DTI tractography and functional imaging should help differentiate between brain regions active during task performance and those activated in response to age-related deterioration [69].

In 2007, a study among normal people in China identified age-related alterations in the white matter of the brain. The main aim of the study was to look into the relationship between cerebral white matter and FA using DTI. The study comprised 45 people aged 25–35 years old (young), 45–55 years old (middle-aged) and 65 and older, all of whom had normal cerebral white matter MRI results. FA was measured in (ROIs) that included the corpus callosum's genu and splenium, the posterior and anterior limbs of the internal capsule, the centrum semiovale, frontal white matter, the thalamus and the head of the caudate nucleus. FA values diminish with age, notably in the genu of the corpus callosum, the centrum semiovale and the frontal white matter, according to the study [70].

A study was carried out in the United States in 2013 to investigate normal brain development using DTI. This narrative review discussed the various diffusivity parameters and their relationship to normal brain development. The purpose of this review is to shed light on the various factors that influence paediatric DTI. White matter anisotropy is minimal in newborn and gradually increases with age. While changes in white matter MD and anisotropy frequently occur at the same time during maturation, with MD values decreasing and anisotropy values increasing, the methods by which the two parameters change are conceptually distinct. Even though there is little known about the relationship between FA and MD changes, they are not always correlated, and a change in one does not always correspond to a change in the other. This study reported the following findings. During development, white matter anisotropy values increase in three stages: fascicle formation, proliferation and maturation of glial cell bodies and intracellular compartments and myelination. Fibre organization occurs primarily in humans while they are still in the womb, as evidenced by anisotropy in late intrauterine and preterm infants. This method should primarily improve anisotropy while having little effect on MD. The initial rise appears to coincide with the developmental growth of immature oligodendrocytes before the histological appearance of myelin. Notably, premyelination is detected as an increase in anisotropy, whereas T1- or T2-weighted imaging does not. The second stage is characterized by the maturation of glial cell bodies and processes, as well as the formation of the cytoskeleton and various intracellular structures, with an increase in anisotropy but a decrease in MD. The third stage is related to the histological development of myelin and its maturation surrounding axons and is marked by a constant rise in anisotropy. Like brain development, this three-stage rise in white matter anisotropy is not synchronous for various brain regions.

There were significant regional differences in white matter FA values. These disparities are usually governed by the "high FA in the core and low FA in the peripheral white matter" rule. First, despite its relatively deep location, the area where the corpus callosum and the anterior limb of the internal capsule connect ("crossing" region) has a low FA at birth and lacks an initial steep FA increase. Second, association fibre maturation, notably in the superior longitudinal fasciculus, occurs later in development. Despite their tiny size, limbic fibres (the fornix and the cingulum) can be seen in the early stages of development. The corticospinal tract is the most developed, followed by the spinothalamic tract and fornix, the arcuate and inferior longitudinal fasciculus, optic radiations and the anterior limb of the internal capsule and the cingulum, according to diffusivity and anisotropy along the pathways in normal-term infants. According to the study, correct knowledge must be obtained by researchers to lay the groundwork for both improving our understanding of normal brain development and exploring the pathophysiological basis of developmental diseases.

Summary: In this chapter, we have introduced the physics and clinical evidence of the most important scalar derivative of DTI: fractional anisotropy. In Chap. 6, we shall be discussing the hardware and instrumentation related to diffusion-tensor imaging.

References

1. Pierpaoli C, Basser PJ. Toward a quantitative assessment of diffusion anisotropy. Magn Reson Med. 1996;36(6):893–906. http://www.ncbi.nlm.nih.gov/pubmed/8946355.
2. Papadakis NG, Xing D, Houston GC, Smith JM, Smith MI, James MF, et al. A study of rotationally invariant and symmetric indices of diffusion anisotropy. Magn Reson Imaging. 1999;17(6):881–92. http://www.ncbi.nlm.nih.gov/pubmed/10402595.
3. Sorensen AG, Wu O, Copen WA, Davis TL, Gonzalez RG, Koroshetz WJ, et al. Human acute cerebral ischemia: detection of changes in water diffusion anisotropy by using MR imaging. Radiology. 1999;212(3):785–92. http://www.ncbi.nlm.nih.gov/pubmed/10478247.
4. Yoshiura T, Wu O, Zaheer A, Reese TG, Sorensen AG. Highly diffusion-sensitized MRI of brain: dissociation of gray and white matter. Magn Reson Med. 2001;45(5):734–40. http://www.ncbi.nlm.nih.gov/pubmed/11323798.
5. Beppu T, Inoue T, Shibata Y, Kurose A, Arai H, Ogasawara K, et al. Measurement of fractional anisotropy using diffusion tensor MRI in supratentorial astrocytic tumors. J Neurooncol. 2003;63(2):109–16. http://www.ncbi.nlm.nih.gov/pubmed/12825815.
6. Basser P, Pierpaoli C. Recollections about our 1996 JMR paper on diffusion anisotropy. J Magn Reson. 2011;213(2):571–2. http://www.ncbi.nlm.nih.gov/pubmed/22152372.
7. Pierpaoli C, Jezzard P, Basser PJ, Barnett A, Di Chiro G. Diffusion tensor MR imaging of the human brain. Radiology. 1996;201(3):637–48. http://www.ncbi.nlm.nih.gov/pubmed/8939209.
8. Lee CEC, Danielian LE, Thomasson D, Baker EH. Normal regional fractional anisotropy and apparent diffusion coefficient of the brain measured on a 3 T MR scanner. Neuroradiology. 2009;51(1):3–9. http://www.ncbi.nlm.nih.gov/pubmed/18704391.

9. Huisman TAGM, Loenneker T, Barta G, Bellemann ME, Hennig J, Fischer JE, et al. Magnetic resonance. Eur Radiol. 2006;16:1651–8.
10. Huisman TAGM, Bosemani T, Poretti A. Diffusion tensor imaging for brain malformations. Neuroimaging Clin N Am. 2014;24(4):619–37. http://www.sciencedirect.com/science/article/pii/S1052514914000732.
11. Hunsche S, Moseley ME, Stoeter P, Hedehus M. Diffusion-tensor MR imaging at 1.5 and 3.0 T: initial observations. Radiology. 2001;221(2):550–6. http://pubs.rsna.org/doi/abs/10.1148/radiol.2212001823.
12. Snook L, Paulson L-A, Roy D, Phillips L, Beaulieu C. Diffusion tensor imaging of neurodevelopment in children and young adults. Neuroimage. 2005;26(4):1164–73. http://www.ncbi.nlm.nih.gov/pubmed/15961051.
13. van Norden AGW, de Laat KF, van Dijk EJ, van Uden IWM, van Oudheusden LJB, Gons RAR, et al. Diffusion tensor imaging and cognition in cerebral small vessel disease. Biochim Biophys Acta Mol Basis Dis. 2012;1822(3):401–7. http://www.sciencedirect.com/science/article/pii/S0925443911000913.
14. Pfefferbaum A, Adalsteinsson E, Rohlfing T, Sullivan EV. Diffusion tensor imaging of deep gray matter brain structures: effects of age and iron concentration. Neurobiol Aging. 2010;31(3):482–93. https://linkinghub.elsevier.com/retrieve/pii/S0197458008001401.
15. Treit S, Chen Z, Rasmussen C, Beaulieu C. White matter correlates of cognitive inhibition during development: a diffusion tensor imaging study. Neuroscience. 2014;276:87–97. http://www.sciencedirect.com/science/article/pii/S030645221301035X.
16. Sexton CE, Walhovd KB, Storsve AB, Tamnes CK, Westlye LT, Johansen-Berg H, et al. Accelerated changes in white matter microstructure during aging: a longitudinal diffusion tensor imaging study. J Neurosci. 2014;34(46):15425–36. http://www.ncbi.nlm.nih.gov/pubmed/25392509.
17. Grieve SM, Williams LM, Paul RH, Clark CR, Gordon E. Cognitive aging, executive function, and fractional anisotropy: a diffusion tensor MR imaging study. AJNR Am J Neuroradiol. 2007;28(2):226–35.
18. Paper O. Normal development of human brain white matter from infancy to early adulthood: a diffusion tensor imaging study. Dev Neurosci. 2015;37(2):182–94.
19. Jun Q, Irvin Y, Paolo T, Yi M, Carissa S, Kang K. Tracking cerebral white matter changes across the lifespan: insights from diffusion tensor imaging studies. J Neural Transm (Vienna). 2013;120(9):1369–95.
20. Zhan L. White matter integrity measured by fractional anisotropy correlates poorly with actual individual fiber anisotropy | Academia.edu. [cited 2014 Jun 27]. https://www.academia.edu/3512971/White_Matter_Integrity_Measured_by_Fractional_Anisotropy_Correlates_Poorly_with_Actual_Individual_Fiber_Anisotropy.
21. de Bruïne FT, van Wezel-Meijler G, Leijser LM, van den Berg-Huysmans AA, van Steenis A, van Buchem MA, et al. Tractography of developing white matter of the internal capsule and corpus callosum in very preterm infants. Eur Radiol. 2011;21(3):538–47. http://www.pubmedcentral.nih.gov/articlerender.fcgi?artid=3032189&tool=pmcentrez&rendertype=abstract.
22. Chang MC, Jang SH. Corpus callosum injury in patients with diffuse axonal injury: a diffusion tensor imaging study. NeuroRehabilitation. 2010;26(4):339–45. http://www.ncbi.nlm.nih.gov/pubmed/20555157.
23. Liu F, Vidarsson L, Winter JD, Tran H, Kassner A. Sex differences in the human corpus callosum microstructure: a combined T2 myelin-water and diffusion tensor magnetic resonance imaging study. Brain Res. 2010;1343:37–45. http://www.ncbi.nlm.nih.gov/pubmed/20435024.
24. Provenzale JM, Isaacson J, Chen S, Stinnett S, Liu C. Correlation of apparent diffusion coefficient and fractional anisotropy values in the developing infant brain. Am J Roentgenol. 2010;195(6):W456–62. http://www.pubmedcentral.nih.gov/articlerender.fcgi?artid=3640803&tool=pmcentrez&rendertype=abstract.
25. Kim EY, Park H-J, Kim D-H, Lee S-K, Kim J. Measuring fractional anisotropy of the corpus callosum using diffusion tensor imaging: mid-sagittal versus axial imaging planes. Korean J

Radiol. 2008;9(5):391–5. http://www.pubmedcentral.nih.gov/articlerender.fcgi?artid=2627217&tool=pmcentrez&rendertype=abstract.
26. Sullivan EV, Rohlfing T, Pfefferbaum A. Longitudinal study of callosal microstructure in the normal adult aging brain using quantitative DTI fiber tracking. Dev Neuropsychol. 2010;35(3):233–56. http://www.pubmedcentral.nih.gov/articlerender.fcgi?artid=2867078&tool=pmcentrez&rendertype=abstract.
27. Rutgers DR, Fillard P, Paradot G, Tadié M, Lasjaunias P, Ducreux D. Diffusion tensor imaging characteristics of the corpus callosum in mild, moderate, and severe traumatic brain injury. AJNR Am J Neuroradiol. 2008;29(9):1730–5. http://www.ncbi.nlm.nih.gov/pubmed/18617586.
28. Huisman TAGM, Loenneker T, Barta G, Bellemann ME, Hennig J, Fischer JE, et al. Quantitative diffusion tensor MR imaging of the brain: field strength related variance of apparent diffusion coefficient (ADC) and fractional anisotropy (FA) scalars. Eur Radiol. 2006;16(8):1651–8. http://www.ncbi.nlm.nih.gov/pubmed/16532356.
29. Hasan KM, Gupta RK, Santos RM, Wolinsky JS, Narayana PA. Diffusion tensor fractional anisotropy of the normal-appearing seven segments of the corpus callosum in healthy adults and relapsing-remitting multiple sclerosis patients. J Magn Reson Imaging. 2005;21(6):735–43. http://www.ncbi.nlm.nih.gov/pubmed/15906348.
30. Jeong HK, Lee S-K, Kim DI, Heo JH. The usefulness of fractional anisotropy maps in localization of lacunar infarctions in striatum, internal capsule and thalamus. Neuroradiology. 2005;47(4):267–70. http://www.ncbi.nlm.nih.gov/pubmed/15806429.
31. Hakulinen U, Brander A, Ryymin P, Öhman J, Soimakallio S, Helminen M, et al. Repeatability and variation of region-of-interest methods using quantitative diffusion tensor MR imaging of the brain. BMC Med Imaging. 2012;12:30. http://www.pubmedcentral.nih.gov/articlerender.fcgi?artid=3533516&tool=pmcentrez&rendertype=abstract.
32. Chou M, Mori S. Effects of b-value and echo time on magnetic resonance diffusion tensor imaging-derived parameters at 1.5 T: a voxel-wise study. J Med Biol Eng. 2012;33(1):45–50.
33. Fox RJ, Sakaie K, Lee J-C, Debbins JP, Liu Y, Arnold DL, et al. A validation study of multicenter diffusion tensor imaging: reliability of fractional anisotropy and diffusivity values. AJNR Am J Neuroradiol. 2012;33(4):695–700. http://www.ncbi.nlm.nih.gov/pubmed/22173748.
34. Murphy ML, Frodl T. Meta-analysis of diffusion tensor imaging studies shows altered fractional anisotropy occurring in distinct brain areas in association with depression. Biol Mood Anxiety Disord. 2011;1(1):3. http://www.biolmoodanxietydisord.com/content/1/1/3.
35. Brander A, Kataja A, Saastamoinen A, Ryymin P, Huhtala H, Ohman J, et al. Diffusion tensor imaging of the brain in a healthy adult population: normative values and measurement reproducibility at 3 T and 1.5 T. Acta Radiol. 2010;51(7):800–7. http://informahealthcare.com/doi/abs/10.3109/02841851.2010.495351.
36. Giannelli M, Cosottini M, Michelassi MC, Lazzarotti G, Belmonte G, Bartolozzi C, et al. Dependence of brain DTI maps of fractional anisotropy and mean diffusivity on the number of diffusion weighting directions. J Appl Clin Med Phys. 2009;11(1):2927. http://www.ncbi.nlm.nih.gov/pubmed/20160677.
37. Bisdas S, Bohning DEE, Besenski N, Nicholas JSS, Rumboldt Z. Reproducibility, interrater agreement, and age-related changes of fractional anisotropy measures at 3T in healthy subjects: effect of the applied b-value. AJNR Am J Neuroradiol. 2008;29(6):1128–33. http://www.ajnr.org/cgi/doi/10.3174/ajnr.A1044.
38. Mandl CW, Schnack HG, Zwiers MP, Van Der SA. Functional diffusion tensor imaging: measuring task-related fractional anisotropy changes in the human brain along white matter tracts. PLos One. 2008;3(11):e3631.
39. Schlu M, Drescher R, Rexilius J, Lukas C, Hahn HK, Przuntek H, et al. Diffusion tensor imaging-based fractional anisotropy quantification in the corticospinal tract of patients with amyotrophic lateral sclerosis using a probabilistic mixture model. AJNR Am J Neuroradiol. 2007;28(4):724–30.
40. Farrell JAD, Landman BA, Jones CK, Smith SA, Prince JL, van Zijl PCM, et al. Effects of signal-to-noise ratio on the accuracy and reproducibility of diffusion tensor imaging-derived

fractional anisotropy, mean diffusivity, and principal eigenvector measurements at 1.5 T. J Magn Reson Imaging. 2007;26(3):756–67. http://www.pubmedcentral.nih.gov/articlerender.fcgi?artid=2862967&tool=pmcentrez&rendertype=abstract.

41. Soriano-Raya JJ, Miralbell J, López-Cancio E, Bargalló N, Arenillas JF, Barrios M, et al. Tract-specific fractional anisotropy predicts cognitive outcome in a community sample of middle-aged participants with white matter lesions. J Cereb Blood Flow Metab. 2014;34(5):861–9. http://www.pubmedcentral.nih.gov/articlerender.fcgi?artid=4013764&tool=pmcentrez&rendertype=abstract.
42. Taylor P, Brander A, Kataja A, Saastamoinen A, Ryymin P, Huhtala H. Acta radiologica diffusion tensor imaging of the brain in a healthy adult population: normative values and measurement reproducibility at 3 T and 1.5 T. Acta Radiol. 2010;51(7):800–7.
43. Giannelli M, Cosottini M, Michelassi MC, Lazzarotti G, Belmonte G, Bartolozzi C, et al. Dependence of brain DTI maps of fractional anisotropy and mean diffusivity on the number of diffusion weighting directions. J Appl Clin Med Phys. 2009;11(1):2927. http://www.jacmp.org/index.php/jacmp/article/view/2927/1797.
44. Zhang Y, Schuff N, Jahng G-H, Bayne W, Mori S, Schad L, et al. Diffusion tensor imaging of cingulum fibers in mild cognitive impairment and Alzheimer disease. Neurology. 2007;68(1):13–9. http://www.pubmedcentral.nih.gov/articlerender.fcgi?artid=1941719&tool=pmcentrez&rendertype=abstract.
45. Papanikolaou N, Karampekios S, Papadaki E, Malamas M, Maris T, Gourtsoyiannis N. Fractional anisotropy and mean diffusivity measurements on normal human brain: comparison between low- and high-resolution diffusion tensor imaging sequences. Eur Radiol. 2006;16(1):187–92. http://www.ncbi.nlm.nih.gov/pubmed/15997366.
46. Qin W, Yu CS, Zhang F, Du XY, Jiang H, Yan YX, et al. Effects of echo time on diffusion quantification of brain white matter at 1.5T and 3.0T. Magn Reson Med. 2009;61(4):755–60.
47. Hui ES, Cheung MM, Chan KC, Wu EX. B-value dependence of DTI quantitation and sensitivity in detecting neural tissue changes. Neuroimage. 2010;49(3):2366–74. http://www.ncbi.nlm.nih.gov/pubmed/19837181.
48. Chung AW, Thomas DL, Ordidge RJ, Clark CA. Diffusion tensor parameters and principal eigenvector coherence: relation to b-value intervals and field strength. Magn Reson Imaging. 2013;31(5):742–7. http://www.ncbi.nlm.nih.gov/pubmed/23375836.
49. Szczepek E, Czerwosz L, Szary C, Czernicki Z. [Diffusion tensor imaging (DTI) in the differential diagnosis of normal pressure hydrocephalus and brain atrophy]. Pol Merkur Lekarski. 2014;37(220):221–6. http://www.ncbi.nlm.nih.gov/pubmed/25518577.
50. Bastin ME, Armitage PA, Marshall I. A theoretical study of the effect of experimental noise on the measurement of anisotropy in diffusion imaging. Magn Reson Imaging. 1998;16(7):773–85. http://www.ncbi.nlm.nih.gov/pubmed/9811143.
51. Koyama T, Marumoto K, Domen K, Ohmura T, Miyake H. Diffusion tensor imaging of idiopathic normal pressure hydrocephalus: a voxel-based fractional anisotropy study. Neurol Med Chir (Tokyo). 2012;52(2):68–74. http://www.ncbi.nlm.nih.gov/pubmed/22362286.
52. Giannelli M, Belmonte G, Toschi N, Pesaresi I, Ghedin P, Traino AC, et al. Technical note: DTI measurements of fractional anisotropy and mean diffusivity at 1.5 T: comparison of two radiofrequency head coils with different functional designs and sensitivities. Med Phys. 2011;38(6):3205–11. http://www.ncbi.nlm.nih.gov/pubmed/21815395.
53. Chepuri NB, Yen Y, Burdette JH, Li H, Moody DM, Maldjian JA. Diffusion anisotropy in the corpus callosum. AJNR Am J Neuroradiol. 2002;23(5):803–8.
54. Marenco S, Rawlings R, Rohde GK, Barnett AS, Robyn A, Pierpaoli C, et al. NIH Public Access. 2007;147(1):69–78.
55. Hunsche S, Moseley ME, Stoeter P, Hedehus M. Diffusion-tensor MR imaging at 1.5 and 3.0 T: initial observations. Radiology. 2001;221(2):550–6. http://www.ncbi.nlm.nih.gov/pubmed/11687703.
56. Jansen JFA, Kooi ME, Kessels AGH, Nicolay K, Backes WH. Reproducibility of quantitative cerebral T2 relaxometry, diffusion tensor imaging, and 1H magnetic resonance spectroscopy at 3.0 Tesla. Invest Radiol. 2007;42(6):327–37. http://www.ncbi.nlm.nih.gov/pubmed/17507802.

57. Löbel U, Sedlacik J, Güllmar D, Kaiser WA, Reichenbach JR, Mentzel H. Diffusion tensor imaging: the normal evolution of ADC, RA, FA, and eigenvalues studied in multiple anatomical regions of the brain. Neuroradiology. 2009;51(4):253–63. http://media.proquest.com/media/pq/classic/doc/1664748221/fmt/pi/rep/NONE?hl=&cit:auth=Löbel,+Ulrike;Sedlacik,+Jan;Güllmar,+Daniel;Kaiser,+Werner+A;Reichenbach,+Jürgen+R;Mentzel,+Hans-joachim&cit:title=Diffusion+te.
58. Bénézit A, Hertz-Pannier L, Dehaene-Lambertz G, Monzalvo K, Germanaud D, Duclap D, et al. Organising white matter in a brain without corpus callosum fibres. Cortex. 2015;63:155–71. http://www.sciencedirect.com/science/article/pii/S0010945214002858.
59. Kochunov P, Thompson PM, Lancaster JL, Bartzokis G, Smith S, Coyle T, et al. Relationship between white matter fractional anisotropy and other indices of cerebral health in normal aging: tract-based spatial statistics study of aging. Neuroimage. 2007;35(2):478–87. http://www.sciencedirect.com/science/article/pii/S1053811906011943.
60. Inano S, Takao H, Hayashi N, Abe O, Ohtomo K. Effects of age and gender on white matter integrity. AJNR Am J Neuroradiol. 2011;32(11):2103–9. http://www.ncbi.nlm.nih.gov/pubmed/21998104.
61. Barrick TR, Charlton RA, Clark CA, Markus HS. White matter structural decline in normal ageing: a prospective longitudinal study using tract-based spatial statistics. Neuroimage. 2010;51(2):565–77. https://linkinghub.elsevier.com/retrieve/pii/S1053811910002016.
62. Yasmin H, Aoki S, Abe O, Nakata Y, Hayashi N, Masutani Y, et al. Tract-specific analysis of white matter pathways in healthy subjects: a pilot study using diffusion tensor MRI. Neuroradiology. 2009;51(12):831–40. http://www.ncbi.nlm.nih.gov/pubmed/19662389.
63. Zhai G, Lin W, Wilber KP, Gerig G, Gilmore JH. Comparisons of regional white matter diffusion in healthy neonates and adults performed with a 3.0-T head-only MR imaging unit. Radiology. 2003;229(3):673–81. http://www.ncbi.nlm.nih.gov/pubmed/14657305.
64. Moon W-J, Provenzale JM, Sarikaya B, Ihn YK, Morlese J, Chen S, et al. Diffusion-tensor imaging assessment of white matter maturation in childhood and adolescence. Am J Roentgenol. 2011;197(3):704–12. http://www.ncbi.nlm.nih.gov/pubmed/21862815.
65. Jones DK. The effect of gradient sampling schemes on measures derived from diffusion tensor MRI: a Monte Carlo study. Magn Reson Med. 2004;51(4):807–15. http://www.ncbi.nlm.nih.gov/pubmed/15065255.
66. Heiervang E, Behrens TEJ, Mackay CE, Robson MD, Johansen-Berg H. Between session reproducibility and between subject variability of diffusion MR and tractography measures. Neuroimage. 2006;33(3):867–77. http://www.ncbi.nlm.nih.gov/pubmed/17000119.
67. Pfefferbaum A, Adalsteinsson E, Sullivan EV. Replicability of diffusion tensor imaging measurements of fractional anisotropy and trace in brain. J Magn Reson Imaging. 2003;18(4):427–33. http://www.ncbi.nlm.nih.gov/pubmed/14508779.
68. Caiazzo G, Trojsi F, Cirillo M, Tedeschi G, Esposito F. Q-ball imaging models: comparison between high and low angular resolution diffusion-weighted MRI protocols for investigation of brain white matter integrity. Neuroradiology. 2016;58(2):209–15. http://www.ncbi.nlm.nih.gov/pubmed/26573606.
69. Sullivan EV, Pfefferbaum A. Diffusion tensor imaging and aging. Neurosci Biobehav Rev. 2006;30:749–61. https://linkinghub.elsevier.com/retrieve/pii/S0149763406000467.
70. Luan P, Hua Q-Q, Lu B-X, Pan S-Y, Zhang X-L. [A diffusion tensor magnetic resonance imaging study of age-related cerebral white matter diffusion anisotropy in normal human adult]. Nan Fang Yi Ke Da Xue Xue Bao. 2007;27(10):1524–7. http://www.ncbi.nlm.nih.gov/pubmed/17959531.

Diffusion-Tensor Imaging Instrumentation

6

The previous chapter briefly described the physics behind the scalar derivative of diffusion-tensor imaging, i.e. fractional anisotropy. The current chapter throws light on DTI instrumentation: hardware and software components for diffusion-tensor imaging. The minimum requirements to achieve acceptable DTI imaging for quantification of FA values at the brain grey and white matter will be discussed in detail. The room layout and design specifications of the MR scan room should be in line with guidelines prescribed by competent MRI authorities worldwide.

6.1 MRI Hardware for Diffusion-Tensor Imaging

The process of acquiring magnetic resonance images consists of a series of controlled processes and coordinated event sequences. However, diffusion-tensor imaging is one of the most recently developed sophisticated neuroimaging techniques available which require advanced MR hardware requirements compared to routine imaging techniques. The major hardware requirements for MR-DTI would include the following as depicted in Fig. 6.1:

1. A strong superconducting magnet
2. A dedicated radio frequency source device
3. An advanced gradient coil system
4. An advanced image processor
5. Highly advanced computer system

R. P. Kotian, P. Koteshwar, *Diffusion Tensor Imaging and Fractional Anisotropy*, https://doi.org/10.1007/978-981-19-5001-8_6

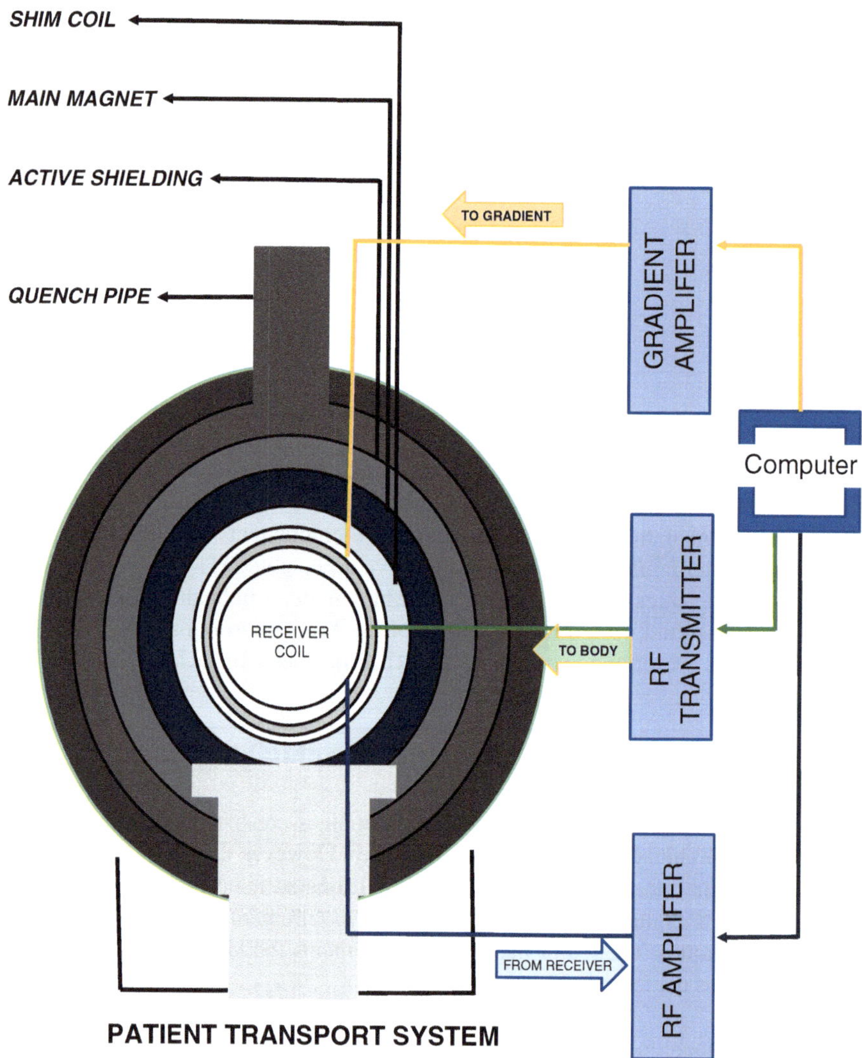

Fig. 6.1 Schematic representation of MRI instrumentation

6.2 Superconducting Magnet Specifications for Diffusion-Tensor Imaging

The invention of superconducting magnet technology in the field of magnetic resonance opened the way for neuroimaging diffusion-tensor imaging and fractional anisotropy. The basic principle lies in using an electromagnet made up of superconducting wire coils which are supercooled to cryogenic temperatures to make it zero electrical resistance. These magnets can produce higher strength magnetic fields [1].

Table 6.1 Magnet system details for diffusion-tensor imaging

Field strength	1.5, 3, 7 or 11.4 T[a]
Bore size	60–70 cm[a]
Magnet length	Min 122–137 cm[a]
Helium consumption	New technology (zero helium boil-off technology)[a]

[a]Implies variations in design for MRI magnets among different vendors

The magnets specially employed in diffusion-tensor imaging belong to Type-1 superconductors which comprise of metals and metalloids showing conductivity at room temperature. The conductor employed in all modern superconducting MR scanners is niobium-titanium showing its superconductivity at 9.4°K. However, scanners employing a magnetic field strength above 10 T utilize a niobium-tin combination. These coils are kept in liquid helium to achieve supercooling to exhibit zero resistivity in a specialized container known as a cryostat where these coils are embedded within a copper core. When compared to the alloy's zero resistance, the surrounding copper core also acts as an insulator at low temperatures [2, 3].

Diffusion-tensor imaging and fractional anisotropy imaging of the brain grey and white matter are possible with superconducting magnets of 1.5 T and higher. Magnets above 1.5 T, namely, 3, 7 T, and the most recent 11.4-T magnets offer superior SNR and spatial resolution in less time. A basic summary of MRI technical magnet details for diffusion-tensor imaging is summarized in Table 6.1.

6.2.1 Gradient Coils for Diffusion-Tensor Imaging

Gradients are coils of wire situated within the bore of the main magnet as depicted in Fig. 6.2. The main purpose of the gradient coil is to alter the strength of the main magnetic field from one end to another by either increasing or decreasing it linearly. This is achieved by passing an electric current through the gradient coils. However, many gradient characteristics contribute to its actual functioning. The change in magnetic field strength relative to its isocentre is determined by the direction of the current to the gradient coil which in turn exhibits its positive or negative polarity. The power of the gradient coils is manipulated using a separate device known as gradient amplifiers. The main functions of gradient coils are as follows:

(a) Slice selection
(b) Frequency encoding
(c) Gradient-echo pulse sequences

Gradient characteristics eventually affect the working principle of gradient coils which in turn causes changes in the main magnetic field. The MR active nucleus' precessional frequency is proportional to the strength of the main magnetic field. As a result, gradient coils are extremely important in MR imaging [4]. The gradient

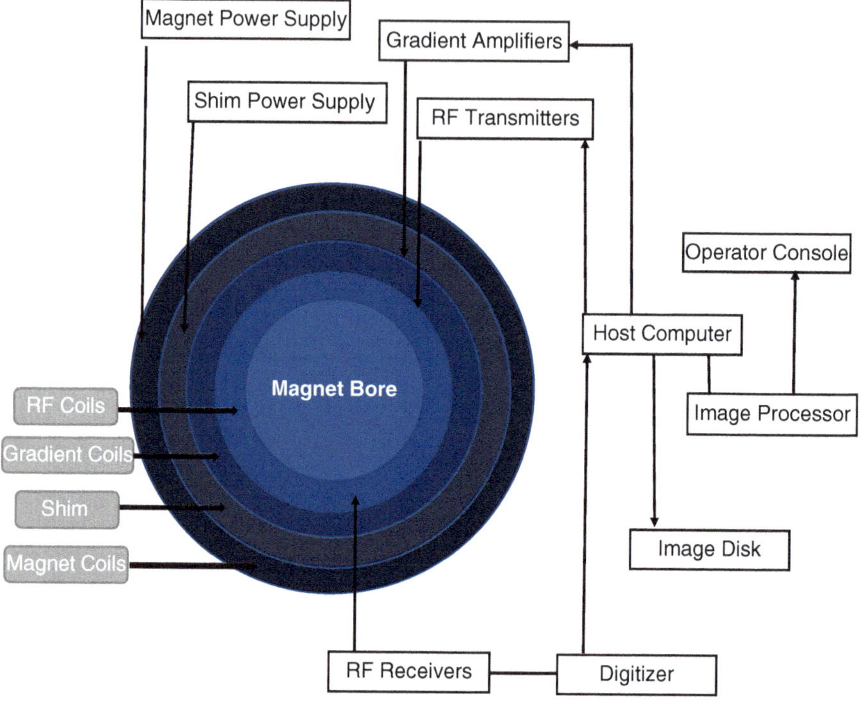

Fig. 6.2 Gradient and RF coil system

Table 6.2 Typical gradient coil system details for diffusion-tensor imaging

Gradient amplitude	28–44 mT/m[a]
Gradient slew rate	95–125 T/m/s[a]

[a]Implies variations in gradient performance characteristics for MRI magnets among different vendors

performance of any MR system will be determined based on the following characteristics, and details of a typical MR scanner system for diffusion-tensor imaging are mentioned in Table 6.2:

(a) **Gradient amplitude (strength)** is the maximum achievable change of magnetic field strength per metre along the bore of the main magnet measured in millitesla per meter (mT/m).
(b) **Gradient speed (rise time)** is the actual time it takes for a gradient coil system to achieve maximum amplitude measured in microseconds (μs).
(c) **Slew rate** is defined as the time it takes for a gradient coil to reach maximum amplitude exhibiting its maximum speed and strength measured in millitesla per meter per second (mT/m/s).
(d) **Duty cycle** is the capacity beyond which the gradients will not be able to work or function and is measured in units of percentage (%).

6.2.2 Radiofrequency Coils for Diffusion-Tensor Imaging

Radiofrequency coils (RF) are referred to as both transmitting and signal receiving devices used in MR imaging [5] and is depicted in Fig. 6.2. RF coils can be broadly classified into the following types:

(a) **Transmit only (body coil within the bore does the duty of transmitting RF)**
The transmit-only coils are usually designed to transmit radiofrequency pulses. The body coil situated within the bore of the magnet is a classic example. These coils are usually coupled with receive coils to receive the MR signals.
(b) **Receive only (e.g. surface coils)**
The receive-only coils are specially designed for small anatomy extremity imaging like the knee, wrist and shoulder joint and only receive MR signals. These coils are coupled with transmit-only coils which emit RF.
(c) **Transmit and receive (e.g. volume coil, head coil, body coil and birdcage quadrature coil)**
This type of coil transmits RF and receives the MR signal simultaneously. These coils provide a good range of FOV for both head and body imaging.
(d) **Phased-array coils (multiple coil elements and channels)**
Phased-array coils consist of multiple coils and receive elements that acquire signals from a particular volume of tissue within the region of interest and combine them all into a single image for improved SNR and coverage [6]. Phased-array coils can be used from a minimum of four coil arrays to up to 204[1] coil elements.

A technical summary of MRI RF coil technology details used for diffusion-tensor imaging is summarized in Table 6.3.

Table 6.3 MRI RF coil technology

*RF technology**	
Number of channels	15–204[a]
Number of independent receiver channels used in a single FOV	10–24, 48, 64[a]
Coil type	8–32-channel head coil with current latest coil technology

*Signifies these numbers vary between manufacturing companies and these specifications undergo constant improvements
[a]Implies variations in RF coil performance characteristics for MRI scanners among different vendors

[1] Signifies these numbers vary between manufacturing companies and these specifications undergo constant improvements.

6.2.3 Shim Coils in Diffusion-Tensor Imaging

One of the most desirable features of any MR scanner would be to create a perfectly homogenous magnetic field for diffusion-tensor imaging and tractography as depicted in Fig. 6.2. However, stringent efforts are being made to ensure a good homogeneity of the main magnetic field by a process known as shimming which utilizes an additional shim coil. The process in which the magnet is shimmed using metal is termed passive shimming, whereas active shimming is achieved by passing an electric current through loops of wire [7, 8]. Diffusion-tensor imaging requires an almost homogenous environment of 0.05–0.5 PPM (parts per million) or less at the centre of the magnetic bore.

6.3 Software Requirements for DTI Applications

FSL, DSI studio, TrackVis, BrainSuit, ExploreDTI, Medinria, PANDA and other DTI software are available on the market for the analysis and quantification of FA values. Each software will have its own set of advantages and disadvantages. A summary of minimum software requirements for diffusion-tensor imaging is outlined in Table 6.4. The basic concept for software requirements for DTI falls under the below-mentioned categories. However different manufacturing companies name them accordingly for their marketing demands and needs.

Table 6.4 DTI software specifications

DTI software requirements*	
Software	Utility
TOPUP	Corrections for susceptibility-related distortions and artefacts
EDDY	Corrections for eddy currents and patient movement
DTIFIT	Used for tensor model fitting and calculating DTI output, for example, FA
FLIRT and FNIRT	Helps in DTI registration to standard image space
TBSS	Used for tract-based localizations, registration, the final output of FA values and comparing FA values between two groups

*Signifies these numbers vary between manufacturing companies and these specifications undergo constant improvements

References

1. Lvovsky Y, Stautner EW, Zhang T. Novel technologies and configurations of superconducting magnets for MRI. Supercond Sci Technol. 2013;26:093001.
2. Maeda H, Yanagisawa Y. Recent developments in high-temperature superconducting magnet technology (review). IEEE Trans Appl Supercond. 2014;24(3):1–12.
3. Budker D, Romalis M. Optical magnetometry. Nat Phys. 2007;3:227–34.
4. Pruessmann KP, Weiger M, Scheidegger MB, Boesiger P. SENSE: sensitivity encoding for fast MRI. Magn Reson Med. 1999;42(5):952–62.
5. Gruber B, Froeling M, Leiner T, Klomp DWJ. RF coils: a practical guide for nonphysicists. J Magn Reson Imaging. 2018;48(3):590–604.
6. Walsh DO, Gmitro AF, Marcellin MW. Adaptive reconstruction of phased array MR imagery. Magn Reson Med. 2000;43(5):682–90.
7. Mao W, Smith MB, Collins CM. Exploring the limits of RF shimming for high-field MRI of the human head. Magn Reson Med. 2006;56(4):918–22.
8. Stockmann JP, Witzel T, Keil B, Polimeni JR, Mareyam A, Lapierre C, et al. A 32-channel combined RF and B0 shim array for 3T brain imaging. Magn Reson Med. 2016;75(1):441–51.

7 Diffusion-Tensor Imaging and Fractional Anisotropy Protocol at 1.5-T MRI for Early Parkinson's Disease

7.1 Introduction: Diffusion-Tensor Imaging Protocol for Obtaining FA at the Brain White and Grey Matter

MRI is a very well-established non-invasive imaging technique that provides the best contrast resolution among the existing diagnostic imaging modalities. MRI has been used as a gold standard for brain imaging involving all neurodegenerative diseases. However, specific neuro-related disorders are still not easily detectable using routine MR imaging. Hence, the use and need of specialized and hybrid imaging techniques must be realized for the early detection of neurodegenerative disorders which are not picked by routine MR imaging techniques. Diffusion-tensor imaging (DTI) is a sophisticated imaging technique that can help in detecting microstructural brain abnormalities. FA values derived from DTI as its scalar derivative can help in predicting early changes and findings over a wide range of neurodegenerative diseases.

Significance of Including the White- and Grey-Matter Regions of the Brain for FA in Early Parkinson's Disease

In the study findings reported in later chapters, the region of interest (ROI) technique was used to calculate FA values at the following white- and grey-matter brain regions: corpus callosum (head, body and splenium), centrum semiovale (right and left), pons (right and left), substantia nigra (three areas), thalamus (right and left), cerebral peduncles (right and left), cerebellar peduncles (right and left), putamen (right and left) and caudate nucleus (right and left). The above-mentioned regions of the white and grey matter of the brain were based on significant clinical evidence reported in the literature on PD where FA values were found useful [1, 2].

R. P. Kotian, P. Koteshwar, *Diffusion Tensor Imaging and Fractional Anisotropy*,
https://doi.org/10.1007/978-981-19-5001-8_7

7.2 Quantitative Factors Affecting DTI and FA Values

As discussed earlier in Chap. 4, FA values have no fixed units and a small range between 0 and 1. To categorize factors affecting FA, we can simply divide them into qualitative and quantitative parameters. The qualitative factors do not affect FA directly compared to its counterpart. Many factors are affecting FA, namely, the magnetic field strength, time of repetition (TR), time of echo (TE), diffusion-weighted directions, type of coil and the homogeneity of the magnet. A greater degree of anisotropic motion will result in higher FA values than its counterpart, which will result in lower FA values. The number of diffusion-weighted directions in an MRI system also influences FA values [3]. The echo time (TE) and *b*-value are two other factors that have a quantitative impact on FA values [4].

b-Value of 1000 is superior to other values and shows good reproducibility in most anatomic locations by studies reported in literature [4]. FA decreases as *b*-value decreases, and FA increases as TE increases [5]. FA values are used to screen, treat and follow up on patients who have neurological abnormalities. Clinical studies have shown that FA values are a reliable predictor of white-matter abnormalities in the elderly and neurological disorders [6].

Studies conducted on *b*-value and time of echo (TE) to check for the accuracy and repeatability of diffusion tensor-derived indices obtained at 1.5 T revealed that both these factors affect results obtained in grey and white matter of the brain [5].

Hence, a detailed DTI protocol mentioning technical and key parameters like combinations of *b*-value and TE will help inaccurate interpretation of FA values. The studies that have been published so far have failed to depict a standard and fixed protocol with *b*-value and TE to obtain consistent FA values.

7.2.1 Specific Indications for DTI in Early Parkinson's Disease

Indications for MR-DTI of the brain mainly include, but are not limited to:

1. Detection of disrupted connections of the dopaminergic pathway [7]
2. Evaluation of the white-matter tracts connecting the substantia nigra and striatum, mainly nigrostriatal tract (NST) [7]
3. Loose Lewy body confined at the medulla oblongata, pontine tegmentum and olfactory bulb/anterior olfactory nucleus [7]
4. Overall brain myelin disruption [8]
5. Overall brain connectivity [8]
6. Overall brain atrophy/putaminal atrophy in particular [8]

7.2.2 General Contraindications for MRI

Contraindications for MR-DTI of the brain mainly include:

1. The presence of an implant that is magnetically or electrically activated (e.g. cardiac pacemaker, artificial heart valves, neurostimulator, cochlear implant and any hearing aids)
2. Clips for intracranial aneurysms and ferromagnetic surgical clips (except for titanium)
3. The presence of a metallic foreign body in the eye
4. Metal or bullets impacting the brain
5. Pregnancy (justify benefit vs. unknown risk to the foetus)
6. Unstable or uncooperative patients or claustrophobia

7.2.3 Patient Preparation for MR-DTI Brain Examination

Patient preparation for MR-DTI brain examination mainly includes:

1. Obtaining written consent from the patient before the start of the MRI scan
2. Removal of any metallic or magnetic objects before entering the scanner room
3. Offering earplugs or sound muffing headphones with a music option
4. Providing a bystander for claustrophobic patients (e.g. relatives or staff)
5. Explaining the MRI brain scan procedure in-depth and stressing the importance of remaining still through the scan time of 10–25 min approximately
6. Lastly, measuring and noting down the accurate weight of the patient

7.2.4 Technical Positioning Considerations for MR-DTI Brain

The following steps should be taken to ensure a good MR-DTI brain scan:

1. Place the patient supine head-first on the MR imaging table.
2. Place the head into the head coil, and use sponges wherever required for accurate packing of the head into the coil avoiding any movement of the head.
3. Use sponges and cushions under the patient's neck and head for accurate positioning accuracy.
4. Give extra cushions under the knee, hips and ankle for extra lower limb comfort.
5. Use Velcro strap in both hands to avoid any upper limb movement
6. Lastly, centre the laser beam localizer over the glabella.

7.3 MR-DTI Protocol for Early PD

Scan parameters	DTI medium sequence for early PD
Magnetic fields	1.5–3 T
Number of $b = 0$ (s/mm^2)	$b = 0$ and $b = 1000$ s/mm^2
Number of directions	15–64 (or more)
Slice thickness (mm)/interval	2, 0 mm

Scan parameters	DTI medium sequence for early PD
Recon voxel size	1.75
TR (MS)	8602
TE (MS)	100
b-Value	1000
Matrix	112 × 110
BW in EPI frequency direction	1781.9
FOV (mm)	224
NEX	3
Diffusion-weighted directions	15
EPI factor	59
Imaging mode	EPI single shot
Flip angle	90°
Fat suppression	SPIR
SAR	≤10%
Parallel imaging	GRAPPA
Average scan time	4–8 min (or longer)

EPI echo-planar imaging, *NEX* number of excitations or signal averages, *SPIR* spectral pre-saturation with inversion recovery, *SAR* specific absorption rate, *GRAPPA* generalized auto calibrating partial parallel acquisition

7.3.1 MRI Conventional Brain Routine Sequences for PD

Images should be captured using a head coil system with at least 16 channels. To rule out neurological abnormalities, conventional imaging (T1-weighted axial and T2-weighted FLAIR axial) should be performed. The technical imaging parameters for T2-weighted FLAIR are as follows: TR/TE/inversion time (TI)/flip angle = 1 1,000 ms/100 ms/2800 ms/180°, slice thickness = 5 mm, number of slices = 40, matrix size = 272 × 180 and field of view (FOV) = 272 × 180 mm. Parameters used for T1-weighted sagittal imaging include the following: TR/TE/flip angle = 500 ms/11 ms/69°, slice thickness = 5 mm, number of slices = 40, matrix size = 292 × 181 and field of view (FOV) = 292 × 181 mm. Conventional MR imaging is one of the prerequisites for DTI. FA values can be computed by overlapping DTI images with T1 sagittal or T2 FLAIR images for anatomical correlation.

7.3.2 DTI-MR Brain Planning for Estimating FA Values

A three-plane localizer should be taken in all three planes in the beginning to plan conventional brain imaging sequences. The T1 sagittal slices are then planned on the axial plane of the localizer with sufficient angulation and the central slice perpendicular and passing through the anterior and posterior commissures. The T2

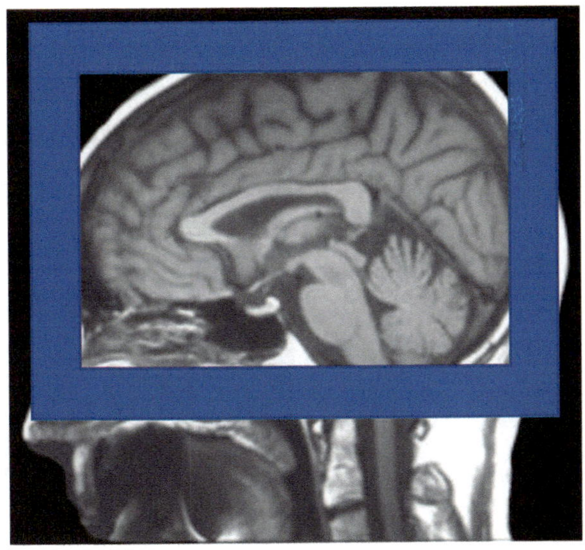

Fig. 7.1 DTI brain planning on T1 sagittal image plane

FLAIR axial slices can now be planned on the T1 sagittal plane parallel to the anterior and posterior commissures. Lastly, the DTI-MR brain planning is done on the T1 sagittal plane as a volume 3D acquisition without any angulation as depicted in Fig. 7.1.

7.3.3 DTI Post-processing for FA Values

The extended MR workspace Philips workstation was used for ROI identification and FA value estimation. To visualize and calculate fractional anisotropy values, the DTI image sets were uploaded alongside routine water suppression sequence FLAIR and T1-weighted sequence for anatomy visualization. ROIs were drawn in the brain white- and grey-matter regions using standard techniques and anatomy reference overlap sequences, as shown in Figs. 7.2, 7.3, 7.4, 7.5, 7.6 and 7.7. The details of the Philips extended MR workspace used for study reports are as follows: Version 2.6.3.1–7.1.5.1 (2009–2017).

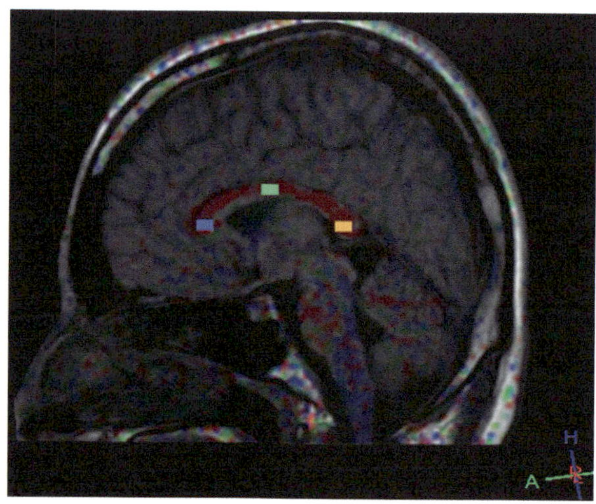

Fig. 7.2 ROI at corpus callosum (genu, body and splenium)

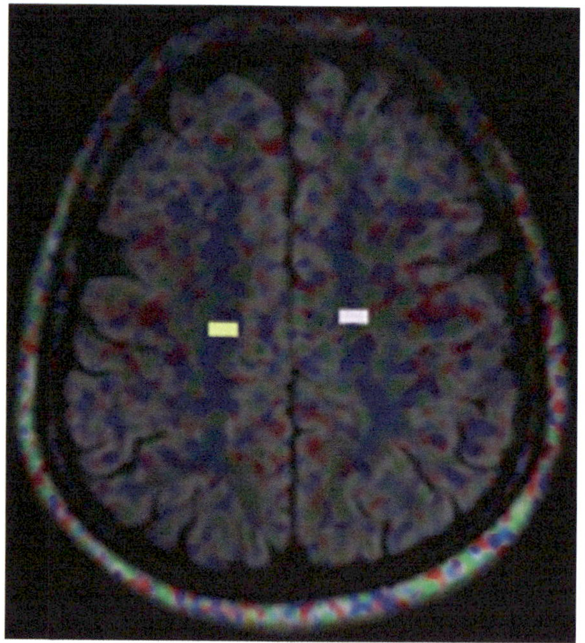

Fig. 7.3 ROI at centrum semiovale (right and left)

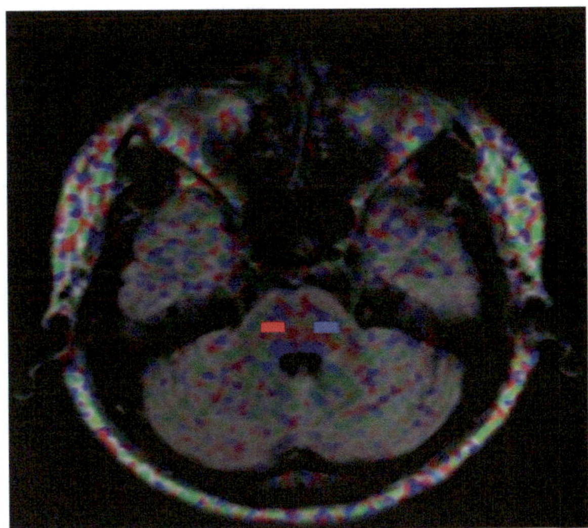

Fig. 7.4 *ROI at the* pons

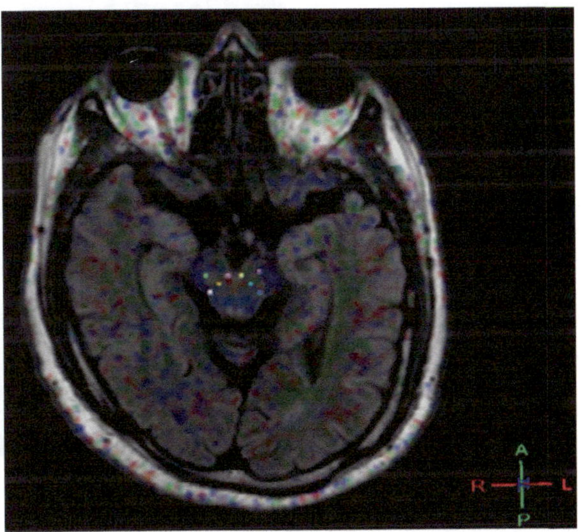

Fig. 7.5 ROI at substantia nigra and cerebral peduncles

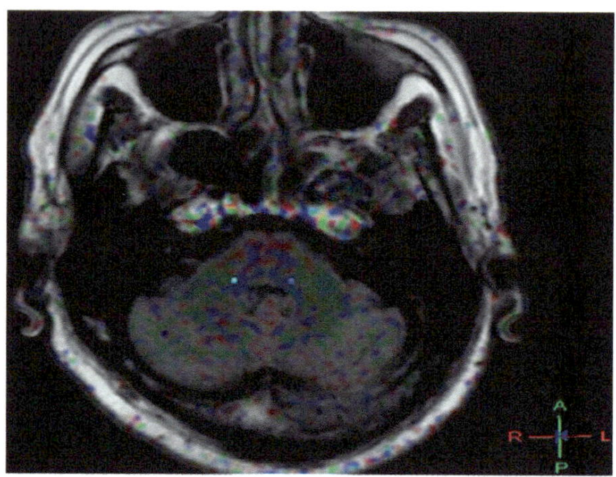

Fig. 7.6 ROI at cerebellar peduncles

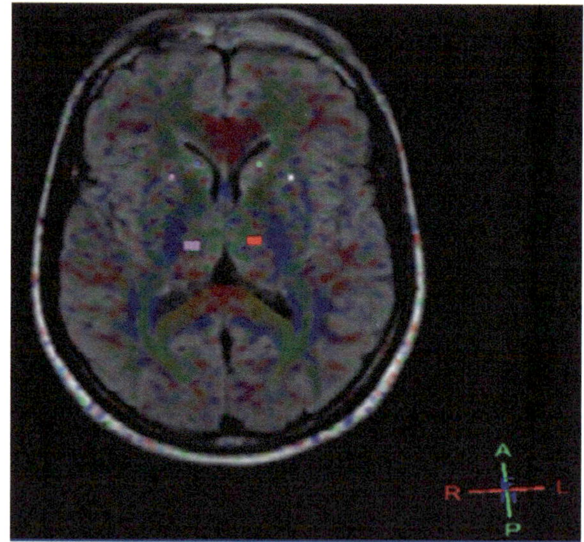

Fig. 7.7 ROI at caudate nucleus, putamen and thalamus

References

1. Cochrane CJ, Ebmeier KP. Diffusion tensor imaging in parkinsonian syndromes: a systematic review and meta-analysis. Neurology. 2013;80(9):857–64.
2. Atkinson-Clement C, Pinto S, Eusebio A, Coulon O. Diffusion tensor imaging in Parkinson's disease: review and meta-analysis. NeuroImage Clin. 2017;16:98–110.
3. Giannelli M, Cosottini M, Michelassi MC, Lazzarotti G, Belmonte G, Bartolozzi C, et al. Dependence of brain DTI maps of fractional anisotropy and mean diffusivity on the number of diffusion weighting directions. J Appl Clin Med Phys. 2009;11(1):2927. http://www.jacmp.org/index.php/jacmp/article/view/2927/1797.
4. Bisdas S, Bohning DEE, Besenski N, Nicholas JSS, Rumboldt Z. Reproducibility, interrater agreement, and age-related changes of fractional anisotropy measures at 3T in healthy subjects:

effect of the applied b-value. AJNR Am J Neuroradiol. 2008;29(6):1128–33. http://www.ajnr.org/cgi/doi/10.3174/ajnr.A1044.
5. Chou M, Mori S. Effects of b-value and echo time on magnetic resonance diffusion tensor imaging-derived parameters at 1.5 T: a voxel-wise study. J Med Biol Eng. 2012;33(1):45–50.
6. Zhang Y, Schuff N, Jahng G-H, Bayne W, Mori S, Schad L, et al. Diffusion tensor imaging of cingulum fibers in mild cognitive impairment and Alzheimer disease. Neurology. 2007;68(1):13–9. http://www.pubmedcentral.nih.gov/articlerender.fcgi?artid=1941719&tool=pmcentrez&rendertype=abstract.
7. Zhang Y, Burock MA. Diffusion tensor imaging in Parkinson's disease and parkinsonian syndrome: a systematic review. Front Neurol. 2020;11:1–25.
8. Heim B, Krismer F, De Marzi R, Seppi K. Magnetic resonance imaging for the diagnosis of Parkinson's disease. J Neural Transm. 2017;124(8):915–64.

Introduction: Types of Parkinson's Disease

8

8.1 Background

Parkinson's disease (PD) is the most popular variety of parkinsonism and is known as "idiopathic parkinsonism" because the cause is unknown. PD is a common neurology-related disorder after Alzheimer's. Reduction of dopaminergic cells and increased iron deposition in the SN of the midbrain are the primary pathophysiologic causes of tremors, bradykinesia and rigidity. Motor symptoms are seen due to loss of dopamine, whereas nonmotor symptoms are through cholinergic, serotoninergic or noradrenergic systems. This neurodegenerative disease is also called a subtype of synucleinopathy. A protein called alpha-synuclein is abnormally accumulated in the brain leading to the destruction of brain cells resulting in PD-specific symptoms. Clinically and pathologically many neurodegenerative diseases mimic each other and the most common being the close resemblance of PD being mimicked as Alzheimer's disease. In Alzheimer's disease, however, a different protein known as tau protein accumulates in brain cells. Thus, clinical presentations differ predominantly, and dementia is the presentation of Alzheimer's disease, whereas tremors and imbalance would be the presentation of PD [1].

Along with a low level of dopamine, a low level of norepinephrine due to the damage of the nerve endings results in both motor and nonmotor symptoms in PD. Lewy body dementia, a type of neurodegenerative disease but not PD, also presents with movement and behaviour abnormalities where dementia is its predominant feature [2]. Another subtype of PD is vascular parkinsonism where a patient presents with symptoms of PD with its pathophysiology being vascular events leading to infarcts involving dopaminergic pathway. Similarly, infection and metabolic causes also can present with PD symptoms [3].

Multiple system atrophy (MSA), dementia (Lewy bodies), progressive supranuclear palsy (PSP) and corticobasal degeneration are all neurodegenerative disorders associated with Parkinson-Plus syndrome. Their collective clinical features overlap, and hence these disorders are called a part of a continuum of PD [4].

R. P. Kotian, P. Koteshwar, *Diffusion Tensor Imaging and Fractional Anisotropy*, https://doi.org/10.1007/978-981-19-5001-8_8

PD is a progressive disease and advances over worsening of symptoms as dopamine levels progressively diminish. It usually appears around the age of 60 and is 50% more common in males than in females. The early-onset disease is found in 10% by the age of 50 itself. Several imaging markers are available, in differentiating PD from PD-Plus and vascular dementia complex. Most of the imaging is advised to upkeep clinical diagnosis by exclusion. Imaging is important to follow up on the progression of the disease and to plan appropriate interventions like deep brain stimulation. To date, diagnostic markers are deficient, and underdiagnosis or misdiagnosis of the condition is still high. As imaging markers, conventional MRI is followed by focused nigrosome imaging, neuromelanin imaging, iron mapping (quantitative) and DTI [4]. CT scan results will be usually normal. MRI might show certain features like loss of swallowtail configuration of substantia nigra, thinning of SN on proton density or T2* sequences. Secondary or compounding causes of parkinsonism, such as encephalitis, chronic ischemic changes and rare causes of basal ganglia tumours and hydrocephalus, are ruled out using CT and MRI scans. PET and SPECT scans in nuclear medicine are used to assess the activity of dopamine transporters in the basal ganglia.

The main scope of this chapter is to outline the role of the DTI matrix in early PD, monitor the benefit of progression of PD and understand the typical region of involvement in atypical PD or PD-Plus syndromes. Review on the correlation of DTI matrix with the evolution of PD where different areas are successively engaged will also be discussed [5].

8.2 DTI Matrix

Various DTI matrices and their significance are described in the previous chapters. The FA and MD are important DTI parameters. A tractogram of white matter gives an overall qualitative and quantitative measure of the fibres. Tractography helps in the visualization of neural connectivity profiles.

FA represents the orientation of water molecule distribution, whereas MD represents water molecule-free diffusion. Thus, FA is an indicator of the integrity of neural tracts and MD represents tissue degeneration. Both these parameters are markers of pathological alteration in brain tissues. FA ranges from 0 to 1. Normal white matter shows the highest anisotropy close to 1, and as degeneration progresses, anisotropy increases and FA value drops [6]. As a result, substantia nigra FA values in Parkinson's disease patients will be significantly lower than in healthy individuals. The SN, the cingulate, corticospinal tract, CC and temporal cortices are very sensitive to FA.

As previously reported, abnormal FA values are detected in PD using DTI before the formation of atrophy, which is then visualized on conventional MRI, implying DTI as a robust imaging biomarker of PD. In the presymptomatic stages of PD, subcortical and sympathetic nervous system degenerations are seen, and as the disease progresses, cortical changes appear [3, 5].

In PD, FA levels are significantly lower in the SN and its surrounding areas. As the disease progresses, subcortical white matter also shows reduced FA upon comparison to a healthy population. However, deep GM nuclei do not show any changes concerning DTI parameters. There might be extrapyramidal site involvement involving the striatal circuit (principal) and its accessory circuits. In PD, accessory circuits involve nigrostriatal projections of the third and fourth circuits which also show significantly low FA irrespective of the duration of PD. Regions under the principal circuit are the thalamus, cortex, neostriatum and globus pallidus [6].

It has been established that approximately half of the dopaminergic cells in the SN are lost after the onset of clinical symptoms in PD. As a result, FA can be used as an imaging marker to predict disease onset and progression in the future. Similarly, when compared to healthy controls, disease progression is associated with a decrease in FA value in the SN. PD also has an impact on the anterior olfactory structures, WM near the gyrus rectus and frontal WM [7].

According to the proven hypothesis, PD prodromal motor symptoms are a late presentation. The main pathology of PD does not begin in the SN; rather, a wide range of nonmotor symptoms precede traditional motor symptoms of PD much earlier. Neurotropic pathogens reach the brain via nasal or oral pathway reaching the olfactory tracts much earlier than substantia nigra resulting in olfactory functional disturbances. It is well-identified that loss of sense of smell is the first feature of appearance in Parkinson's disease, occurring a decade or more before the onset of motor symptoms. As a result, there is a greater risk of developing PD in a population with olfactory disturbances [8].

Rather than direct changes in the olfactory epithelium, pathophysiology describes the deposition of Lewy body protein in various areas of the olfactory territory [7]. The olfactory bulb is one of the primary regions of the brain to be affected by PD. Thus, DTI findings in the gyrus rectus and the WM involving primary olfactory areas are well documented. The olfactory tracts travel on the inferior surface of the frontal lobe and are located in the olfactory grooves. They then split distally into medial-intermediate to lateral striae. Technical challenges due to susceptibility artefacts from the sinuses are high in the post-processing of tractography which also lacks evidence-based results. Especially with PD patients, there will be neuronal loss and disruption within the bundle, and it is much more difficult to derive tractography of an olfactory system when compared to healthy individuals. It is worth mentioning that olfactory disorders are also seen in sinonasal polyposis which is much more prevalent than PD and thus conventional MRI should be done to rule out polyposis before labelling the patient as early PD [8].

In general, reduced FA and increased MD suggest demyelination or degeneration of cells with increased extracellular space. However, corticospinal tract shows an increase in FA and reduction in MD representing some amount of reorganization of brain cells. Concerning diagnosis and progression of PD, varied results are found in the literature with mixed findings of both increase and decrease in FA compared to the control group. Exposure to certain chemicals for >20 years was considered a predefined risk factor for PD. With this background, few studies also tried to show that FA was a sensitive enough tool in identifying the population at risk when compared to healthy population [9].

White-matter changes also correlate with the dementia component of PD. Dementia will be found in many later stages and is indicative of chronic advanced PD. Thus, FA increase and MD decrease in white-matter genu are linked to PD dementia and attention dysfunctions [10, 11]. Cognitive impairment can be graded as normal, mild or dementia by the DTI matrix, especially with FA and MD values in the body and splenium of corpus callosum [12]. Structural alteration of these regions also correlates with gait disorders [13]. Thus, corpus callosum involvement in PD is an indicator of the advanced stage of the PD [14]. Internal and external capsule degenerations are potential additional markers of Parkinson's disease that are highly correlated with clinical UPDRS motor score and gait disturbance [15, 16].

The corticospinal tract has an increase in FA and a decrease in MD, indicating reorganization of fibres or increased axonal activity or axonal sprouting as a compensatory mechanism for decreased input from the thalamus and striatum. The cause for corticospinal FA increase might be due to significant neurodegeneration because of *altered* pallido-thalamic activity [17].

Few studies tried to correlate FA value in subcortical nuclei with patients' symptoms. They tried to identify FA in subcortical nuclei when symptoms like tremor "off" or dyskinesia "on" and concluded that DTI matrix changes are related to bradykinesia, cognitive status and level of dopamine [5].

"A very few studies also derived the results of medication-induced alteration in midbrain GM volume (SN, tegmental ventral area and subthalamic nucleus) but not DTI" [18, 19]. "Levodopa and iron chelation therapy would have intrinsic magnetic properties and might misregister signal intensity of GM and thus wrongly classify GM and WM volume". This concept needs to be further studied to strengthen the evidence [18–20].

DTI of the putamen and pallidum is not very consistent in uniform results. FA changes are insignificant in putamen and pallidum suggesting sparing of these regions by Parkinson's disease [21–23]. Caudate nucleus shows an increase in FA but no change in MD values suggesting a reorganization of cells [24]. Interestingly, it has been established that cognitive dysfunction in PD is caused by damage to the temporal and cingulate cortices. These regions show reduced FA and increased MD values suggesting temporal cortex degeneration is the cause of the cognitive decline of PD group [12, 25]. DTI can also be used to investigate microstructural changes brought about by specific training [26, 27] and has been proposed to demonstrate reorganization of specific areas in certain human pathologies [28] and animal models [29].

8.3 Comparing FA Values of PD with Other Neurodegenerative Diseases

PSP: According to a study that partitioned the CC, reduced FA in CC1 (prefrontal region) may differentiate PSP from PD, with receiver operating characteristic analysis demonstrating the reliability of FA (85.7% sensitivity, 65.5% specificity and 69.4% accuracy). DLB patients have lower FA in various white-matter regions such as the dorsal striatum, amygdala, inferior longitudinal fasciculus, corpus callosum, frontoparietal and occipital regions, which is a late feature or is not frequently seen in Parkinson's disease. DTI measurements were used by Prodoehl et al. to critically compare patients with Parkinson's disease from healthy controls and patients with essential tremor and Parkinson-Plus syndromes. FA in the posterior SN was substantially higher in healthy controls than in early tremors, PD, MSA-P and PSP patients. In addition, FA in the posterior caudate was lower in MSA-P patients compared to PSP patients. DTI measurements managed to perform well in identifying patients with Parkinson's disease from those with other parkinsonian syndromes, with sensitivity and specificity ranging from 90 to 100%. Pyatigorskaya et al. recently discovered that NM-based SN volume and FA in the pons were the best predictors of differentiating PSP from PD using multimodal nigral imaging. According to the results of this study, multimodal nigral imaging is a promising tool for assessing neurodegeneration in PSP patients [30, 31].

To summarize, a handful of studies have compared the presence of WM abnormalities in DLB patients to healthy controls or other neurodegenerative diseases. In DLB patients, DTI revealed extensive structural connectivity abnormalities, including decreased FA in various cerebral regions such as CC, dorsal striatum, parietal, frontal, occipital, amygdala and lastly inferior longitudinal fasciculus [1]. More research is needed, however, because no specific pattern has been identified.

8.4 Diffusion Tensor Imaging: Tumours (Neoplastic and Non-neoplastic Lesion Characterization with DTI)

DTI-derived FA values can be a reliable strategy for surgeons in planning their surgical approach to reduce the surgical risk and to improve surgical outcomes. Pre-op and intra-op DTI can help surgeons in better tumour delineation with preservation of neurological functions. Applications of DTI in characterization, knowing the extent of intracranial tumours and differentiating neoplastic from non-neoplastic lesions are well demonstrated. Tubercular infection is considered one of the closest mimickers of many intracranial neoplasms. "Many lesions show a similar pattern of peripheral ring enhancement on conventional MRI commonly depicting tubercular granuloma, metastasis and a few gliomas" [32, 33]. DTI is also very helpful in differentiating abscess vs. necrotic neoplastic lesions and highly cellular lesions like lymphoma from low cellularity tumours like glioma. It is also useful in distinguishing tumour recurrence from pseudoprogression and vasogenic oedema from tumour-infiltrated oedema. Other applications include differentiation between suckable from non-suckable tumours depending on FA value in pituitary adenoma vs. meningioma. Pituitary adenoma would show low FA compared to meningioma, thus indicating a very soft tumour and amenable for sucking. DTI gives valuable information about the tract's infiltration and displaced course as a result of the tumour and is thus recognized as an essential tool for preoperative surgical planning.

Brain tumours are prominently found in or near areas of eloquence, such as motor and language areas. These tracts are frequently injured during surgical resection of such tumours, resulting in severe neurologic complications. It is critical to have a preoperative understanding of the tumour's relationship to the tract [33].

The FA is the most widely used quantitative DTI analysis parameter, representing the percentage of anisotropy in water molecules to total dispersion movement. The FA value ranges from 0 to 1, with 0 indicating isotropic dispersion, which means that the probability and distance of dispersion in all directions are equal, and 1 indicating a high degree of directional dependence of the dispersion motion of water molecules.

The FA, mean diffusivity (MD) and colour-coded structural diffusion tensor maps are gaining clinical importance recently. FA can be measured by placing the ROI within the lesion. Further characterization of the type of tumour is possible by the assessment of perilesional oedema, within 1 cm from tumour margin and also the ratio of FA in tumour to normal white matter. Tractography images are of great utility in directly visualizing the adjacent white-matter tracts and their relation with the tumour. Tracts are divided into three types: displaced, infiltrated and disrupted. Displacement occurs when the tract exhibits an abnormal location and/or direction but has normal or only slightly decreased FA. Reduced anisotropy which remains identifiable on the colour map is defined as infiltrated. Isotropic diffusion with a non-identifiable tract on the directional colour map is called disrupted [34].

Perilesional oedema differs in primary neoplastic when compared to metastatic brain lesions. Perilesional oedema of glioma contains infiltrating glial tumour cells and increased aquaporin-4 expression, whereas capillaries or cells resemble the organ of origin in cases of oedema surrounding metastasis.

Soni et al. compared 25 glioma ad 25 cases of non-neoplastic cases. The perilesional MD was higher for the non-neoplastic group compared to the neoplastic group with statistical significance; however, lesional MD was statistically insignificant. FA of oedema and lesion was higher in the neoplastic group compared to the non-neoplastic group, however not statistically insignificant. The lesional FA was statistically higher in tuberculomas compared to metastases but no perilesional oedema. However, differentiation of the non-neoplastic group from tuberculoma by DTI parameters within the lesion and perilesional oedema was not possible.

FA decides the integrity and density of white-matter fibres, and MD depends on the degree of vasogenic oedema. Mean diffusivity characterizes the presence of hindrances to diffusion, and fractional anisotropy is related to the intactness of oriented white-matter fibres. Gliomas present with more white-matter fibre destruction and less vasogenic oedema in comparison with non-neoplastic lesions; thus, a higher perilesional MD favours a non-neoplastic pathology [34].

FA has a limited role in grading tumours from high to low grade as FA values are inconsistent. Features like increased vascularity, oedema, the presence of micro-cysts and larger tumour cell sizes decrease FA which is representative of high-grade tumours according to the WHO [35].

8.5 Surgical Extent and Outcome vs. DTI and Tractography

Preoperative mapping of cortical regions and functionally relevant WM tracts is aided by DTI. It directs the surgeon to have a greater extent of resection (EOR) while also reducing post-operative deficits. Tractography provides information about the tumour proximity, impactness and invasion of WMT. Assertive resection of DTI abnormalities was associated with a higher chance of survival [36].

Lower FA and higher MD in the affected hemisphere's cerebrospinal tract (CST), as well as a distance of <8 mm from the tumour margin to the CST, result in post-operative motor deficits. Preservation of the arcuate fasciculus and superior longitudinal fasciculus, for example, results in good long-term language function. Preserving interhemispheric connectivity reduces aphasia. Injury to optic radiation can be avoided by the use of DTI mapping generated preoperatively [37–40].

Intraoperative DTI (iDTI) tractography is also possible in the present era. The reliability of preoperative iDTI depends on physiological brain shift, which causes deformation. These may be caused by CSF drainage, tumour collapse, swelling, resection and drugs. Marongiu et al. investigated the post-operative outcomes of tumour resections that were accompanied by iDTI. EOR was significantly higher with iDTI (88.5% vs. 44%) and 6-month survival was higher (73.1% vs. 38.9%) [41].

Other modes of assessment of tumour extent intraoperatively are sparse data-driven biomechanical model, navigated ultrasound of direct in-organ contact and Doppler to enable blood vessel visibility. Combing direct electrical stimulation (DES) with DTI will help in more focused stimulation. The more the proximity with tracts, the lower the required stimulation current, thus reducing hemodynamic changes across large areas of the brain. Functional MRI along with tractography adds knowledge of the functionality of tracts even when tracts are not visualized through tractography like in cases of significant infiltration. Tractography ability is limited in deriving multiple fibres and also due to the partial volume effect. Higher-order diffusion models, such as kurtosis imaging (DKI), constrained spherical convolution (CSD) and generalized Q-ball imaging (GQI), are now available. Further evidence by research is yet to be accomplished to bring DTI into clinical utility specifically in tumour grading and differentiating post-operative recurrence vs. treatment changes [42].

References

1. Bae YJ, Kim JM, Sohn CH, Choi JH, Choi BS, Song YS, et al. Imaging the substantia nigra in Parkinson disease and other Parkinsonian syndromes. Radiology. 2021;300(2):260–78.
2. Lenfeldt N, Larsson A, Nyberg L, Birgander R, Forsgren L. Fractional anisotropy in the substantia nigra in Parkinson's disease: a complex picture. Eur J Neurol. 2015;22(10):1408–14.
3. Karagulle Kendi AT, Lehericy S, Luciana M, Ugurbil K, Tuite P. Altered diffusion in the frontal lobe in Parkinson disease. AJNR Am J Neuroradiol. 2008;29(3):501–5.
4. Tessa C, Giannelli M, Della Nave R, Lucetti C, Berti C, Ginestroni A, et al. A whole-brain analysis in de novo parkinson disease. AJNR Am J Neuroradiol. 2008;29(4):674–80. http://www.ncbi.nlm.nih.gov/pubmed/18184843.
5. Atkinson-Clement C, Pinto S, Eusebio A, Coulon O. Diffusion tensor imaging in Parkinson's disease: review and meta-analysis. NeuroImage Clin. 2017;16:98–110. https://doi.org/10.1016/j.nicl.2017.07.011.
6. Report S. Early pathological changes in the parkinsonian brain demonstrated by diffusion tensor MRI. J Neurol Neurosurg Psychiatry. 2004;75(3):481–4.
7. Cochrane CJ, Ebmeier KP. Diffusion tensor imaging in parkinsonian syndromes: a systematic review and meta-analysis. Neurology. 2013;80(9):857–64.
8. Nigro P, Chiappiniello A, Simoni S, Paolini Paoletti F, Cappelletti G, Chiarini P, et al. Changes of olfactory tract in Parkinson's disease: a DTI tractography study. Neuroradiology. 2021;63(2):235–42.
9. Du G, Lewis MM, Sterling NW, Kong L, Chen H, Mailman RB, et al. Microstructural changes in the substantia nigra of asymptomatic agricultural workers. Neurotoxicol Teratol. 2014;41:60–4.
10. Zheng Z, Shemmassian S, Wijekoon C, Kim W, Bookheimer SY, Pouratian N. DTI correlates of distinct cognitive impairments in Parkinson's disease. Hum Brain Mapp. 2014;35(4):1325–33.
11. Kamagata K, Tomiyama H, Motoi Y, Kano M, Abe O, Ito K, et al. Diffusional kurtosis imaging of cingulate fibers in Parkinson disease: comparison with conventional diffusion tensor imaging. Magn Reson Imaging. 2013;31(9):1501–6.
12. Deng B, Zhang Y, Wang L, Peng K, Han L, Nie K, et al. Diffusion tensor imaging reveals white matter changes associated with cognitive status in patients with Parkinson's disease. Am J Alzheimers Dis Other Demen. 2013;28(2):154–64.
13. Chan LL, Ng KM, Rumpel H, Fook-Chong S, Li HH, Tan EK. Transcallosal diffusion tensor abnormalities in predominant gait disorder parkinsonism. Parkinsonism Relat Disord. 2014;20(1):53–9.
14. Hawkes CH, Del Tredici K, Braak H. Parkinson's disease: a dual-hit hypothesis. Neuropathol Appl Neurobiol. 2007;33(6):599–614.
15. Vercruysse S, Leunissen I, Vervoort G, Vandenberghe W, Swinnen S, Nieuwboer A. Microstructural changes in white matter associated with freezing of gait in Parkinson's disease. Mov Disord. 2015;30(4):567–76.
16. Lenfeldt N, Holmlund H, Larsson A, Birgander R, Forsgren L. Frontal white matter injuries predestine gait difficulties in Parkinson's disease. Acta Neurol Scand. 2016;134(3):210–8.
17. Mole JP, Subramanian L, Bracht T, Morris H, Metzler-Baddeley C, Linden DEJ. Increased fractional anisotropy in the motor tracts of Parkinson's disease suggests compensatory neuroplasticity or selective neurodegeneration. Eur Radiol. 2016;26(10):3327–35.
18. Salgado-Pineda P, Delaveau P, Falcon C, Blin O. Brain T1 intensity changes after levodopa administration in healthy subjects: a voxel-based morphometry study. Br J Clin Pharmacol. 2006;62(5):546–51.
19. Chung JW, Burciu RG, Ofori E, Shukla P, Okun MS, Hess CW, et al. Parkinson's disease diffusion MRI is not affected by acute antiparkinsonian medication. NeuroImage Clin. 2017;14:417–21.
20. Campbell N, Hasinoff B. Iron supplements: a common cause of drug interactions. Br J Clin Pharmacol. 1991;31(3):251–5.

21. Menke RAL, Szewczyk-Krolikowski K, Jbabdi S, Jenkinson M, Talbot K, Mackay CE, et al. Comprehensive morphometry of subcortical grey matter structures in early-stage Parkinson's disease. Hum Brain Mapp. 2014;35(4):1681–90.
22. Nagae LM, Honce JM, Tanabe J, Shelton E, Sillau SH, Berman BD. Microstructural changes within the basal ganglia differ between Parkinson disease subtypes. Front Neuroanat. 2016;10:17.
23. Rajput AH, Voll A, Rajput ML, Robinson CA, Rajput A. Course in parkinson disease subtypes: a 39-year clinicopathologic study. Neurology. 2009;73(3):206–12.
24. Hou Y, Yang J, Luo C, Ou R, Song W, Liu W, et al. Patterns of striatal functional connectivity differ in early and late onset Parkinson's disease. J Neurol. 2016;263(10):1993–2003.
25. Carlesimo GA, Piras F, Assogna F, Pontieri FE, Caltagirone C, Spalletta G. Hippocampal abnormalities and memory deficits in Parkinson disease: a multimodal imaging study. Neurology. 2012;78(24):1939–45.
26. Sagi Y, Tavor I, Hofstetter S, Tzur-Moryosef S, Blumenfeld-Katzir T, Assaf Y. Learning in the fast lane: new insights into neuroplasticity. Neuron. 2012;73(6):1195–203.
27. Engvig A, Fjell AM, Westlye LT, Moberget T, Sundseth Ø, Larsen VA, et al. Memory training impacts short-term changes in aging white matter: a longitudinal diffusion tensor imaging study. Hum Brain Mapp. 2012;33(10):2390–406.
28. Yu Z, Tao L, Qian Z, Wu J, Liu H, Yu Y, et al. Altered brain anatomical networks and disturbed connection density in brain tumor patients revealed by diffusion tensor tractography. Int J Comput Assist Radiol Surg. 2016;11(11):2007–19.
29. Ding G, Jiang Q, Li L, Zhang L, Zhang ZG, Ledbetter KA, et al. Magnetic resonance imaging investigation of axonal remodeling and angiogenesis after embolic stroke in sildenafil-treated rats. J Cereb Blood Flow Metab. 2008;28(8):1440–8.
30. Aguiar LP, da Rocha PA, Morris M. Therapeutic dancing for Parkinson's disease. Int J Gerontol. 2016;10(2):64–70.
31. Whitwell JL, Schwarz CG, Reid RI, Kantarci K, Jack CR, Josephs KA. Diffusion tensor imaging comparison of progressive supranuclear palsy and corticobasal syndromes. Parkinsonism Relat Disord. 2014;20(5):493–8. http://www.sciencedirect.com/science/article/pii/S135380201400039X.
32. De Belder F, Van Cauter S, Van Den Hauwe L, Van Hecke W, Emsell L, De Belder M, et al. DTI in diagnosis and follow-up of brain tumors. In: Diffusion tensor imaging: a practical handbook. New York: Springer; 2016.
33. Potgieser ARE, Wagemakers M, van Hulzen ALJ, de Jong BM, Hoving EW, Groen RJM. The role of diffusion tensor imaging in brain tumor surgery: a review of the literature. Clin Neurol Neurosurg. 2014;124:51–8. http://www.sciencedirect.com/science/article/pii/S0303846714002133.
34. Soni N, Srindharan K, Kumar S, Bhaisora KS, Kalita J, Mehrotra A, et al. Application of diffusion tensor imaging in brain lesions: a comparative study of neoplastic and non-neoplastic brain lesions. Neurol India. 2018;66(6):1667–71.
35. Louis DN, Ohgaki H, Wiestler OD, Cavenee WK, Burger PC, Jouvet A, et al. The 2007 WHO classification of tumours of the central nervous system. Acta Neuropathologica. 2007;114(2):97–109.
36. Costabile JD, Alaswad E, D'Souza S, Thompson JA, Ormond DR. Current applications of diffusion tensor imaging and tractography in intracranial tumor resection. Front Oncol. 2019;9:426.
37. Yan JL, Van Der Hoorn A, Larkin TJ, Boonzaier NR, Matys T, Price SJ. Extent of resection of peritumoral diffusion tensor imaging-detected abnormality as a predictor of survival in adult glioblastoma patients. J Neurosurg. 2017;126(1):234–41.
38. Castellano A, Bello L, Michelozzi C, Gallucci M, Fava E, Iadanza A, et al. Role of diffusion tensor magnetic resonance tractography in predicting the extent of resection in glioma surgery. Neuro Oncol. 2012;14(2):192–202.

39. Shiban E, Krieg SM, Haller B, Buchmann N, Obermueller T, Boeckh-Behrens T, et al. Intraoperative subcortical motor evoked potential stimulation: how close is the corticospinal tract? J Neurosurg. 2015;123(3):711–20.
40. Javadi SA, Nabavi A, Giordano M, Faghihzadeh E, Samii A. Evaluation of diffusion tensor imaging-based tractography of the corticospinal tract: a correlative study with intraoperative magnetic resonance imaging and direct electrical subcortical stimulation. Neurosurgery. 2017;80(2):287–99.
41. Marongiu A, D'Andrea G, Raco A. 1.5-T field intraoperative magnetic resonance imaging improves extent of resection and survival in glioblastoma removal. World Neurosurg. 2017;98:578–86.
42. Wang Y, Zhang H, Wang Y, Lu T, Qiu B, Tang Y, et al. Differences between generalized q-sampling imaging and diffusion tensor imaging in the preoperative visualization of the nerve fiber tracts within peritumoral edema in brain. Neurosurgery. 2013;73(6):1044–53.

Evidence of Fractional Anisotropy in Parkinson's Disease

9

9.1 Background

The previous chapter discussed the diffusion-tensor imaging protocol for obtaining consistent region-wise FA at the brain grey matter (GM) and white matter (WM). This chapter will examine the role of FA in Parkinson's disease (PD), including clinical evidence and correlation.

The human brain is comprised of various types of neurons, and its complicated axon arrangement makes it one of the most complex structures in our body. For noninvasively imaging the entire brain in vivo, MRI is one of the safest and easiest medical imaging tools. Conventional MRI may struggle to image the complex axonal structure organization of the brain, whereas DTI, which was introduced in the mid-1990s, has very well understood this complex structure [1]. The findings of numerous animal experimental trials have resulted in DTI being used in routine clinical practice [2]. DTI has a large and diverse set of applications. The main ones are the effective use of DTI in detecting high diffusion anisotropy in unmyelinated nerves [3]. DTI can also detect anisotropy changes in the brain during development without the need for surgery [4, 5]. DTI is effective in detecting pathology in premyelinated brain fields [4]. Animal studies have demonstrated the use of DTI in the phenotype characterization of WM tracts [6]. DTI could be used to explore WM parcellation and connectivity as well [7].

FA value is a scalar derivative of DTI that is being used to express in vivo water diffusion in various directions. The diffusion-tensor data serve as the foundation for calculating eigenvectors or eigenvalues. Many parameters derived from eigenvectors are thus used for anisotropy quantification. FA is currently the best technique for measuring diffusion anisotropy and is widely used in fibre tracking fields [8, 9].

DTI is a method that is increasingly being used in clinical settings to investigate WM and GM integrity in the brain. It is one of the most sophisticated and recently developed neuroimaging techniques for quantifying water diffusion properties

R. P. Kotian, P. Koteshwar, *Diffusion Tensor Imaging and Fractional Anisotropy*,
https://doi.org/10.1007/978-981-19-5001-8_9

in vivo. It can also assess the integrity of microstructures in the brain's WM. Furthermore, DTI is a rapidly evolving and relatively new method for identifying focal lesions in the WM tract in both clinical practice and research. DTI is the only imaging technique that can detect Brownian water movement as it moves through the brain. Diffusion that occurs equally in all directions is said to be isotropic, as opposed to diffusion that is restricted by a barrier, which is said to be anisotropic. FA is the most commonly used diffusion parameter derived from DTI [10]. FA is the best technique for determining diffusion direction, with values ranging from 0 to 1, with 0 indicating isotropic diffusion and 1 indicating elevated anisotropic diffusion. Despite the widespread use of DTI imaging techniques, there are only a few reports that have assessed normative FA values [11–23].

FA values range from 0 to 1 and have no specialized units. High FA values will be reflected by a greater degree of anisotropic motion. FA is also affected by the number of weighting directions for the diffusion [24]. The *b*-value and echo time (TE) are two other factors that influence FA values. FA decreases as *b*-value decreases, and FA increases as TE increases [13]. The two parameters that quantitatively affect FA are TE and *b*-value, among other factors that may also affect them [17]. FA can be used to monitor, treat and track neurological abnormalities. FA values have been shown in clinical studies to be a reliable predictor of white matter abnormalities in ageing and neurological disorders [11]. The *b*-value and TE are the most important factors influencing FA values because they have a quantitative influence on changes in FA.

9.2 Clinical Use of FA in the Brain

A study conducted in 2013 revealed that FA depends on several factors to be clinically significant in medicine and suggested longitudinal imaging studies of white matter structure for assessing fibre orientation and its associated eigen- and FA values [25]. Research on premature infants disclosed a powerful connection between FA and age for fibres connected through the posterior end of the splenium of the CC [26]. The utility of DTI and FA values was proven to be very helpful in identifying injuries to the CC [27]. FA also showed significant variation in males in contrast to females within the genu of the CC, whereas other diffusivity parameters did not show any significant variations [28].

A study conducted on the correlation of ADC and FA values on the developing infant brain revealed that age played an important role in the characterization between these two parameters [29]. A similar study on the CC found that FA on sagittal DTI was higher than FA on axial DTI, and FA obtained from sagittal DTI was more accurate than FA obtained from axial DTI [30]. A research finding on the corpus callosum's adult ageing brain showed that FA in elder adults is lower than in younger adults [16]. The use of DTI in traumatic brain injury was used to detect vasogenic oedema in the genu more than in the splenium of the CC [31]. Different MRI field strengths (i.e. 1.5 and 3 T) show alteration in FA and ADC values, and values on 3 T showed statistically significant values [13]. A study conducted on all normal seven segments of the CC in healthy patients showed gender-independent FA heterogeneity, while patients suffering from multiple sclerosis showed decreased FA values [32]. FA maps and values were found to be very useful in detecting lacunar lesions in different regions of the CC [33]. Variation has been seen in different ROI-based methods, and circular ROI gives a better and higher repeatability rate compared to the freehand ROI [34]. A study conducted on *b*-value and time of echo (TE) to check for the accuracy and repeatability of diffusion tensor-derived indices obtained at 1.5 T revealed that both these factors affect results obtained in grey and white matter [9]. A study conducted on different 3-T magnets and higher angular resolution pulse sequences concludes that FA is the most comparable and reliable parameter than individual diffusivity parameters [35]. A similar study on DTI found a decrease in FA values in the superior longitudinal fasciculus (left), which is useful in detecting depression abnormalities [36]. A study conducted on FA and ADC showed regional variation in different areas of the WM of the brain [37]. The number of diffusion-weighted directions affects FA values, and this study recommended undertaking group and longitudinal studies using the same DTI schemes with fixed directions [38].

A study conducted on developing an infant's brain concluded that FA and ADC values have a strong influence on the aged [29]. The effect of *b*-value on FA has been studied, and it shows that a *b*-value of 1000 is most reproducible in all areas of the brain and FA values change with different *b*-values [39]. A study conducted on the 3-T MR system on 20 regions of the brain showed that FA and ADC do not show a positive correlation between FA and age. It also states that field strength makes a slight difference in the measured FA values [11]. Functional DTI with task activation showed significant changes along white matter neural tracts of the brain [40]. A study conducted with a new DTI quantification model for fibre integrity showed FA values in the corticospinal tract with a high reproducibility [41]. The effects of SNR on diffusion tensor-derived FA values concluded that a minimum set threshold is a must for good and accurate DTI contrast at 1.5 T [42]. Another study conducted revealed that different values of DTI like ADC, RA, FA and eigenvalues revealed that RA is more accurate for age-related structural changes compared to FA [43].

Limited studies are reported in the literature on normative FA at the brain GM and WM. To summarize, FA is a potential imaging tool for detecting neurodegenerative disorders of the brain.

9.3 FA's Role in Parkinson's Disease

PD is a widespread neurodegenerative disorder, and yet its early diagnosis is often far postponed in the course of the disease, and present treatments do not alter the development of the disease. Sixty to 70% of dopaminergic neurons may already be damaged at the time of clinical diagnosis. Thus, early diagnosis and objective measures of disease progression are of utmost importance in developing disease-modifying therapies. Early detection of PD allows clinicians to treat patients and improve their well-being and prognosis. Because PD develops slowly in the brain, standard MRI scans fail to notice any specific changes. Although routine brain MRI scans can detect age-related and atrophy changes, their overall diagnostic utility in PD is low. Structural brain MRI findings are usually normal in PD cases, and the role of MRI in PD has been strictly to rule out its secondary causes. Because laboratory tests fail to detect this disease, UPDRS and the Hoehn and Yahr (H-Y) Scale are the accepted universal techniques for diagnosing PD.

Brain tissue pathology may be reflected in one or more of the following DTI-derived measures: (1) FA; (2) axial diffusivity (AD): the water diffusivity along the primary eigenvector direction; (3) radial diffusivity (RD): the water diffusivity perpendicular to the primary eigenvector direction; and (4) mean diffusivity (MD): the mean water diffusivity along with all directions. Recently, DTI has been successfully applied to detect PD-induced brain tissue abnormalities in multiple grey and white matter regions, and the robust technology has been the use of FA values. Among the few published meta-analyses on DTI and PD are the reported clinical significant findings related to PD. Studies mainly focused on the substantia nigra, a hallmark structure whose degradation is linked to motor symptoms of PD. However, few meta-analyses assessed subcortical, cortical, WM and cerebellar regions and observed significant alterations in PD in many regions including the SN, caudate, putamen, globus pallidus, olfactory cortex and WM at the CC and corticospinal tracts (CST). In most existing studies, DTI measures were obtained from PD patients in Braak's stage 3 or higher. As a result, the reported findings, which might reflect the combination of PD pathology, medication effects and neural compensatory mechanisms at later PD stages, are not highly consistent. For example, (1) DTI measures of the substantia nigra have been variable concerning whether significant differences exist or not between PD patients and controls. (2) A peculiar study conducted in 2016 observed FA increase in some brain regions (e.g. corticospinal tract) and FA decrease in other regions (e.g. uncinate fasciculus) in PD patients, suggesting that tissue in different brain regions may be structurally modulated by PD with distinct pathologically compensatory mechanisms [44]. FA variations in the olfactory tract between early-stage PD patients and tract-based spatial statistics (TBSS) were also recorded [45], implying that DTI signal abnormalities reflecting pathological processes in early PD stages may be clinically detectable. A potential concern regarding studies reported on PD in literature is that the chosen TBSS methods utilized in all studies could be over-conservative and thus potentially susceptible to false negatives, due to the nature of voxel-based analyses or residual image misalignment across the subjects. For these reasons, in a more recent TBSS-based study, only AD difference was observed, but no FA difference, in the olfactory tract between PD and controls [46]. In another comparable research, the writers measured DTI signals from two sets of ROIs (olfactory region; substantia nigra) and discovered that olfactory region DTI signals could better distinguish PD patients from healthy controls compared to substantia nigra signals [46–48]. These issues may be better addressed using advanced DTI processing pipelines, which were recently developed, based on machine learning or tractometry analysis [49, 50].

The present trend of using DTI as a diagnostic instrument in PD has made our knowledge of the structural anomalies underlying PD and its associations with grey and white brain matter important [51]. Although regular brain MRI scans can identify age-related degenerative changes, their diagnostic accuracy in PD is low. Structural brain MRI findings are usually normal in PD cases, and the role of MRI in PD has been strictly to rule out its secondary causes.

The primary aim of this chapter is to explore the function of DTI imaging in various brain areas using FA values in early PD. We shall also recognize the brain areas and their correlation with FA values in PD patients in both GM and WM.

9.4 FA Evidence as Imaging Markers in PD

Structural brain MRI findings are usually normal in PD cases, and the role of MRI in PD has been strictly to rule out its secondary causes. Clinicians must detect PD early to address and enhance the quality of life and survival rate. The latest development of using DTI as a screening tool in PD has emphasized our understanding of structural abnormalities underlying PD and their associations with brain GM and WM, and the use of DTI has been an efficient approach for the PD imaging [51].

FA is one of the most commonly used quantitative measures of diffusion in the brain in PD patients. Changes in FA values have been reported in several PD cases, but the clinical use of DTI in intervention continues to be a challenge [52–56]. Many non-motor symptoms appear years before other symptoms of PD. Because of its dynamic contrast resolution and non-ionizing capability, MRI is presently the best imaging tool for early PD screening.

DTI is an advanced imaging technique to visualize and differentiate diffusion properties in the neurological diseases [1, 10]. Brain tissue abnormalities can be depicted in one or more of the following DTI-derived measures: (1) FA, (2) axial diffusivity (AD), (3) radial diffusivity (RD) and (4) mean diffusivity (MD). Among the following DTI derivatives, FA is found to be the most robust and reliable technique in the brain and to detect its abnormalities held [35, 57]. DTI has recently been shown to be useful in detecting PD in both GM and WM regions of the brain. Till date, three detailed reviews on PD using DTI have been published [58–60]. Two studies focused mostly on substantia nigra (SN) and its association to other clinical presentations of PD [59, 61]. While the third focused on subcortical, cortical, WM and cerebellar areas, it found significant PD changes in vital areas, including the SN, caudate, putamen, globus pallidus, olfactory cortex, CC WM and corticospinal tracts [60]. In most existing studies, the DTI measures were obtained from PD patients in Braak's stage 3 or higher. Hence, the reported findings are a combination of PD pathology, medication effects and neural compensatory mechanisms at later PD stages. For example, the DTI measures at the substantia nigra show inconsistent results whether differences exist or not between PD and control group [59, 60, 62]. Some studies find an increase in FA in some regions (e.g. corticospinal tract) and FA decrease in other regions (e.g. uncinate fasciculus) in PD patients which suggests that FA value in PD will vary based on different regions of the brain [44]. Some studies employ the tract-based spatial statistics (TBSS) technique for DTI data analysis, but some have reported false negatives when using this technique [45, 46, 63, 64].

9.5 Case Reports and Case Series on PD-FA, Corpus Callosum and PD

Wiltshire et al. (2010) conducted a study on the CC and cingulum using DTI in PD subjects in Canada. The study's main goal was to measure FA and MD in the CC and cingulum pathways using DTI in patients with PD and PD with dementia and normal controls and to correlate these measures with mental status scores in PD patients. PD patients who met the criteria for idiopathic PD were included, and those with atypical PD or incidental stroke were excluded. Patients with PD with dementia (PDD) had parkinsonism first and then developed dementia as defined by DSM-IV criteria. All patients and controls underwent the mental status test (MMSE) for cognitive evaluation and finally, PD severity was assessed using the Unified Parkinson's Disease Rating Scale. Image acquisition was done using a 1.5-T Siemens system with conventional imaging including MPRAGE sequence and T2 axial and FLAIR sequences. DTI sequence with standard *b*-value = 1000 s/mm^2, TE = 88 ms and TR = 5600 ms and six diffusion directions were used. Four regions of the CC and two regions, namely, right and left, of the cingulum were evaluated using tractography. Over the specified area of interest, cingulum values were averaged. Analysis of variance was used to compare the various groups studied. When there were group differences, post hoc comparisons were performed using the Bonferroni correction. The intra-rater reliability of measurements was determined using a two-way mixed model with an absolute agreement and single measure interclass correlation coefficients. There was no difference in age between groups, nor was there any difference in the CC or cingulum pathways. MMSE scores in Parkinson's disease patients correlated well with MD in the CC, which was independent of age, gender and white matter volume. The study revealed that the CC or its connections are linked to cognitive impairment in PD patients. There were some suggestions for larger studies in cognitively impaired PD patients that could reveal WM pathology, for example, Parkinson's disease dementia with Lewy bodies [65].

In Sweden, a study was carried out to determine the utility of DTI in PD using a new method to normalize diffusion data. Furthermore, the use of DTI for additional diagnosis in selected white matter tracts was evaluated. Subjects included were 38 PD patients and 16 healthy controls and sub-classified into 10 idiopathic PD (IPD), 16 patients with progressive nuclear palsy (PSP) and 12 patients with multiple system atrophy (MSA). The healthy controls had no history of underlying psychiatric or neurological disease. Image acquisition was done using a 3-T Philips eight-channel head coil. An EPI single-shot sequence with 48 directions, *b*-value = 800 s/mm^2, was used for DTI image acquisition. The regions included in the study were the MCP, cingulum, CST and the CC sections (CC). Whole-brain tractography using multiple areas of interest (ROIs) was done to obtain FA values. To label the difference in groups in patient demographic and categorical data, Fisher's test was used. The Kruskal-Wallis test was used to compare the average FA, MD, RD and apparent area coefficient values (AAC) in the three groups studied. CST in the MSA and PSP groups, CC in the PSP group and cingulum in the PSP group all showed significant changes in DTI parameters. When PSP patients were compared to controls, significant changes were observed in the anterior CC in MD, RD and FA values; CST with MD values; and cingulum with AAC values. The study concluded that the anterior portion of the CC is a promising region for detecting neurodegenerative changes in PSP patients, as well as for differentiating PSP from IPD. The small sample size and manual ROI placement were the study's limitations. The author urged large-scale studies to validate research findings and determine whether DTI can detect diffusion changes in PD in its early stages [66].

A normative study on FA was carried out in the Czech Republic in the year 2013 using a new non-linear colour lookup table (LUT). After estimating normative FA in different regions of the brain, WM were calculated in 76 healthy volunteers, and later its clinical utility was checked in three groups, namely the PD, MSA and healthy volunteers, using 30 and 12 motion probing gradients in 59 subjects. A colour code was assigned to each region of the brain using either green, red or blue colour. FA calculation was done using ROI measurements at the following regions of the brain using a 1.5-T MRI unit: CC, grey matter (precentral gyrus and thalamus), basal ganglia (BG), pyramidal tract and cerebellar peduncles. DTI protocol used for image acquisition was as follows: 10 and 30 gradient directions ($b = 1100$; TR = 8839/8800 ms, TE = 95/98 ms, NEX = 2; matrix = 1,286,128; FOV = 280 mm; GRAPPA = 2 and isotropic voxel size 2.2 mm). For FA value calculations, DTI images were processed offline using FSL. For FA values in the CC, frontal GM, BG and thalamus, the LUT was created using population means and 95% prediction intervals. Clinical utility was seen on 17 MSA patients, 13 PD patients and 17 healthy subjects. Four blinded radiologists classified the subjects as MSA or non-MSA. Using only the LUT in distinguishing MSA subjects from PD subjects and controls, high sensitivity (80%) and specificity (84%) were achieved. The LUTs produced by 12 and 30 MPG were comparable, and FA can be used for clinical diagnosis if properly interpreted. As a result, the study concluded with the generation of a LUT based on normative data. Despite differences in SNR, the LUT was applied to two datasets with different sequence parameters, yielding similar results. The application to MSA was indeed significant guidance for future us.

The study also suggested that using LUT in combination with other imaging techniques could enhance diagnosis in all neurodegenerative disorders, not just MSA [67].

9.6 FA, Substantia Nigra and PD

Aquino et al. [68] conducted a study on the region, substantia nigra (SN) in PD patients in which the volume area, MD, FA and iron concentration were measured, in early (EPD) and late (LPD), in Italy for correlation with clinical scores. The study laid down the following inclusion criteria for PD patients as diagnosis of IPD in accordance to the British PD Society Brain Bank criteria, disease duration of 3–5 years for early PD (EPD) and late PD (LPD) of 6–10 years, UPDR III under therapy, age group 50–75 years, dopamine medication with successful control of motor symptoms, Hoehn and Yahr stage III or less, on treatment and Milan Overall

Dementia Assessment score of 90/100 or more. The inclusion criteria included 42 patients with an equal number of LPD and EPD patients and 20 controls (mean age 61 ± 7.26 years) for comparison. Exclusion criteria included whether patients present rest tremors during MRI scan, motor complications, and jejunal levodopa and if they were under deep brain stimulation treatment. Image acquisition was done using a 1.5-T Siemens unit with conventional sequences MPRAGE, GRE Multiecho, T2W, double echo PD and DTI spin-echo sequence with *b*-value 1200 s/mm^2, TE = 100 ms and TR = 9200 ms with 64 diffusion directions. Especially two inversion recovery sequences were used to highlight the SN area. SN, MD and FA measurements were computed using Basser's method. Polygonal ROI was used on both SN using axial sections. Analysis was done using ANOVA, and the difference between the groups was labelled using Bonferroni corrected non-paired *t*-test. Coming to results, concerning EPD and control group, the LPD SN area was reduced. In EPD, significant area is reduced compared to controls and also between EPD and LPD. ANOVA failed to show any significant differences in MD and FA values. The only limitation quoted was the small sample size [68].

A study conducted in Japan primarily focused on the early pathological changes in PD demonstrated by DTI. The study's main goal was to see if FA was reduced in the SN and nigrostriatal projections of PD patients. FA values in the extrapyramidal area of 12 PD patients and 8 age-matched normal controls were compared. The caudate head, nucleus ventralis lateralis, subcortical WM of the premotor cortex, SN, subthalamic nucleus and lower part of the globus pallidus, putamen and caudate nucleus were all used as regions of interest. The DTI protocol obtained with the 1.5-T unit was as follows: 230 × 230-mm field of view; matrix 128 × 128 with SENSE; SENSE reduction factor = 2, TR/TE = 6000/88; flip angle = 90; two *b*-values (0 and 800 s/mm^2); 36 slices; and 3/0-mm slice/gap. Diffusion sensitization was performed in six different directions. Patients with PD had significantly lower FA in the SN and the lower part of the putamen/caudate complex, according to the findings. Finally, the study concluded that FA in the basal ganglia correlates with an early PD diagnosis. Longitudinal studies on FA and PD were also suggested by the authors [69].

9.7 FA, White and Grey Matter of the Brain and PD

A study was performed on a new tract-based DTI technique to check for changes in the cerebellar hemispheres in PD disease. The study included 16 patients with PD with a mean length of disease of approximately 11 years. The 16 controls included subjects without any history of neurodegenerative disease (7M, 9F; mean age 60.1 ± 7.2 years), and subjects were excluded if any lesions were found on T2W and flair sequences. Imaging was done using a 3-T Siemens 32-channel head coil. Conventional imaging was performed using Sagittal 3D T1 MPRAGE, T2-weighted turbo spin-echo and 3D FLAIR sequence. DTI image acquisition was done using an EPI sequence with *b*-value = 1000 s/mm^2, TR = 6919 ms, TE = 87 ms and used 60 gradient diffusion directions. The regions studied for FA values were cerebellar peduncles and cerebellar hemispheres. The quantitative analysis based on fibre analysis of cerebellar peduncles and cerebellar hemispheres was carried out with DTI software to achieve tract amount, tract length, mean track quantity, FA and ADC. The following statistical tests were used for analysis: Kolmogorov-Smirnov test, the statistical influence was evaluated using means of two samples, one-tailed test and finally equality of variance using Zemen's test. The study revealed a statistically substantial drop of FA in PD patients' cerebellar hemispheres compared to healthy controls. The reported limitation was the use of tractography itself and the small sample size. Larger studies in a larger population should be conducted in the future to look for FA reduction in the cerebellar region, which could be a hint at the decline of cerebellar function in PD [70].

Chin Song et al. (2016) conducted a study to test the diagnostic performance and efficiency of DTI in subjects with PD compared to normal brains in Taiwan. The potential case-control study consisted of 126 PD patients and 91 controls. All anti-Parkinson's drugs were stopped 12 h before the MRI scans to avoid any confounding effects of drugs. The following tests were also done in PD patients: Schwab and England activities test, UPDRS, modified Hoehn and Yahr and finally MMSE. They were excluded if they had any brain abnormalities including hydrocephalus, intracranial surgery and major physical or neuropsychiatric disorders. Imaging was done using a 3-T unit using a 12-channel head matrix coil. DTI was done using a spin EPI sequence with TE = 108 ms, TR = 5700 ms, *b*-value = 1000 s/mm^2, and the total number of diffusion-weighted directions was 30 (non-collinear directions). Conventional imaging was performed using T2-W SE, T2-W FLAIR and T1-W sequences to rule out gross disorders. DTI FA value analysis and image post-processing were done using a specialized Camino software. It was then used to standardize and parcel DTI images into 90 cerebral areas using the automated anatomy (labelling) method. The assumption between disease severity and DTI index was investigated using Pearson's correlation coefficient test. When FA was compared with MD values, the counterpart showed a statistically significant difference. FA showed high and low values across different regions of the brain. Overall, PD patients had higher MD in multiple cortical regions beyond the basal ganglia when compared to controls. Maximum values of MD were found in the ipsilateral middle temporal gyrus. The study concluded that using DTI data might be clinically useful in the future for assessing PD patients. Future DTI studies need to be explored to find the association between dementia in patients with PD [71].

A study was conducted in China to analyse DTI indices in the brain among PD patients. The study's primary objective was to explore abnormal cerebral WM diffusion and its connection to the olfactory tract in PD patients. A special technique called the voxel-based analysis was used that could identify the changes of diffusion in the entire brain unlike the region of interest (ROI) technique. The study employed 25 PD patients according to the UPDRS diagnostic criteria. The disease duration was in the range of 2–30 years. The H&R stage was between 1 and 3 in all patients. The selection of less serious patients was merely to avoid moving during the scan process. Patients with WM lesions due to ischemic changes were excluded from the study. Another group of 25 age- and sex-matched healthy subjects was chosen as control. None of the normal controls had any neurological and psychiatric diseases. MRI acquisition was done using a 3-T Siemens Magnetom with 12 channels and employed a phased-array head coil. The DTI sequence used was an EPI with parallel imaging with a b-value = 1000 s/mm^2, TE = 87 ms and TR = 6000 ms, and FA and MD for the whole brain were calculated. An FSL software package was used to process DTI data. The two-sample student's t-test was used to find differences in FA and MD between two groups, and multiple linear regression was used to estimate the associations between olfactory test scores and DTI parameters with disease duration. The study discovered increased MD in the corticofrontal cortices where olfactory tracks are located in the PD group. When it comes to FA values, they showed a significant correlation in a cluster of left medial cerebellum WM and right rectus gyrus, whereas MD showed a negative correlation between MD values in the right cerebellum's WM. The study concluded that there was a disruption in cerebellar WM in PD patients, which could play a significant role [51].

In 2013, a study on brain WM integrity and cognition in PD was conducted in Norway using DTI. The utility of DTI was evaluated for (a) decreased WM integrity in non-demented PD, (b) decreased WM integrity in PD and early Alzheimer's disease (AD) and (c) cognitive performance in non-demented PD. The study included 18 non-demented PD patients, 18 patients with cognitive disorders due to AD and 19 controls. MRI was performed using a 1.5-T Siemens unit. Three-dimensional T1-weighted image (MPRAGE) sequence axial fluid-attenuated inversion recovery was acquired as routine imaging protocol. DTI sequence was acquired using an EPI sequence with the following parameters: b = 650–750 s/mm^2, 12 diffusion directions, TR = 6100 ms, TE = 117 ms and slice thickness: 3 mm (gap 1.9 mm). TBSS was used to analyse FA values. One-way ANOVA, the Kruskal-Wallis test, the student t-test and the Mann-Whitney test were used to compare the three groups as appropriate. When compared to NC, the study's findings revealed significant differences in DTI in WM at the temporal, parietal and occipital cortex. In the primary region of interest analyses, no significant differences were found between the PD and AD groups, but there was a natural inclination for more anterior changes in AD versus more posterior changes in PD compared to NC. In PD patients, there were significant correlations between DTI parameters in the WM underlying the prefrontal cortex and executive and visuospatial abilities. The study concluded that reduced WM integrity was seen in non-demented PD at the temporal, parietal and occipital cortices. As a result, DTI may be an imaging marker in early PD, and WM changes are linked to cognitive deficiencies in PD. The study's limitations included limited sample size and the use of longitudinal cohort studies to determine the relationship between cognition changes and the early PD [72].

A study was conducted in 2013 to check the utility of DTI and correlate it to Parkinson Rating Scale. The brain areas involved in PD remains unclear, and the utility of DTI remains challenging. In this study, DTI was used to investigate phenotype and its correlation with clinical rating scales. Sixty-four patients were investigated at baseline and followed up for 1, 3 and 5 consecutive years. Mean, radial, axial and FA values were correlated with phenotype and clinical scales using multivariate or univariate analysis correction. The following regions of interest were included: CC genu and splenium, frontal WM, the entrance of capsula externa, caput nucleus caudatus, globus pallidus, putamen, SN, thalamus, pontine nuclei and MCP. The scores for UPDRS-I, UPDRS-II, UPDRS-III, HY scale and the Schwab and England scale were evaluated. The DTI protocol used for image acquisition using a 1.5-T unit was as follows: TR = shortest, TE = 77 ms, flip angle = 90°, field of view = 230 × 230 mm, acquisition matrix = 96 × 96, reconstruction matrix = 256 × 256, b = 1100 s/mm^2, number of gradients = 6 and 24 slices, slice thickness = 3.5 mm and no gaps. The study's findings showed that, except for the UPDRS-III, all rating scales were significantly correlated with diffusion measures. The putamen, globus pallidus and thalamus, in particular, showed higher diffusion as scores worsened.

The researchers concluded that altered diffusion in the thalamus and lentiform nucleus, most likely due to decreased neuronal integrity, is an important factor in explaining differences in clinical performance in PD. The study reported the number of dropout patients as its major limitations [73].

A study was conducted in the Netherlands in 2015 to understand the diagnostic utility of 3-T MRI and DTI in early PD. The primary goal was to see if ROI measures improved 3-T brain MRI diagnostic accuracy in distinguishing between atypical PD and early PD. A cohort of 60 patients with early PD and an initial undetermined diagnosis was studied. Patients were examined by a brain MRI first, followed by routine follow-up. To investigate differences in MD and FA values, DTI data were subjected to TBSS and ROI analysis. The DTI protocol employed was as follows: SS-SE EPI, b-values 0 and 1000 s/mm^2, TR/TE = 13,005/103 ms, diffusion directions = 30, FOV = 240 mm and voxel size 2 × 2 × 2 mm. The following regions of interest were placed: midbrain, putamen, centrum semiovale, the body of CC, external capsule, midbrain, superior cerebellum and superior cerebellar peduncles. The statistical tests used for data analysis were ANOVA and ROC. The study discovered significantly higher MD in the atypical PD group at the CS, body CC, putamen, external capsule, midbrain, superior cerebellum and superior cerebellar peduncles. ROI measures of MD did not affect the diagnostic accuracy of brain MRI in identifying atypical PD. There were a few limitations identified in the study: limited sample size, variation in MD and FA values when using different MR systems and field strengths, lack of follow-up and no correlation with post-mortem cases [74].

A study was conducted in Japan in the year 2012 to check the DTI-derived FA values obtained at different centres for identical humans. FA is a robust tool for moderate changes in water diffusion, but it is affected by parameters like motion probing gradients, SNR and so on. As a result, the study's goal was to assess the inter-centre variability of FA. The study included five healthy volunteers who underwent BTI brain screening thrice at three different scan centres using a 1.5 T having different motion probing gradient schemes. The FA values were compared from the three centres measured at the splenium of the CC, genu of the CC, putamen, posterior limb of the internal capsule, cerebral peduncle, optic radiation and middle cerebellar peduncle. The study found a statistically significant difference between FA values obtained at different scanners and centres. Hence, the study concluded that FA values were affected by using different scanners with different motion probing gradients. These factors have to be looked into when using FA for clinical diagnosis and comparison [75].

In the United Kingdom, a systematic review on DTI in parkinsonian syndromes was conducted in 2013. The study's main objective was to assess the potential of DTI measures in parkinsonian syndromes to identify an imaging biomarker. The authors compiled DTI studies on parkinsonian syndromes and related dementias through databases like Embase and Medline. Of 333 study results, 43 were found useful for inclusion. The most noteworthy finding was lower FA in the SN in PD patients vs. normal controls (−0.639, 95% confidence interval −0.860 to −0.417, $p < 0.0001$). The study concluded that DTI could be a strong biomarker in PD syndromes and suggested that longitudinal studies using FA be conducted to obtain other relevant imaging biomarkers [61].

In 2013, a Swedish study used MR tractography to evaluate regional diffusion changes along WM tracts in PD disorders. The study's main goal was to determine the utility of DTI in parkinsonian disorders. The study included four groups of subjects: those with MSA, PSP, IPD and healthy controls. A 3-T unit was used to obtain DTI with whole-brain coverage. DTI was performed using EPI with 48 diffusion directions (*b*-values 0 and 800 s/mm^2), and a voxel size of 2 × 2 × 2 mm was used. FA values were extracted at the following vital brain areas: CC, CG, CST and MCP. DTI changes at the CST (MSA and PSP), CC (PSP) and CG were found to be statistically significant in the study (PSP). The statistical analysis discovered significant differences in the anterior CC FA values of PSP patients versus controls. According to the findings of the study, DTI can be used to demonstrate specific changes in WM in PD disorders. The anterior portion of the CC can be used effectively to detect changes in PSP patients, as well as to differentiate PSP from IPD. The following limitations were identified in the study: For the FA calculation, a small number of patients and manual ROI placement were used [66].

9.7.1 Variables and Learning Definition Terms

9.7.1.1 Diffusion-Weighted Imaging

DWI is an MR imaging technique that utilizes specific sequences to study the diffusion of water molecules using software to generate images with contrast in MR images. The random motion of molecules within a cell is reflected by its diffusion property known as Brownian motion [76]. Water in its pure state exhibits isotropic diffusion and moves freely in all directions in an environment without restriction. A special quantity known as diffusion coefficient is used to define diffusion in restricted areas [77].

9.7.1.2 *b*-Value

b-Value can be defined as an extrinsic contrast parameter and can be altered by the operator depending upon the pulse sequence used. The sensitivity of any MRI sequence is directly linked to the number of phase movements imposed by diffusion gradients. This movement is calculated or represented using a parameter known as *b*-value or diffusion attenuation [78]. *b*-Values depend mainly on three parameters: gradient interval, strength and duration. The unit used to represent the *b*-value is seconds per square millimetre (S/mm^2). There are two extremes of *b*-values, i.e. high and low. The low value is 0 while the high value is in the range of 1000.

9.7.1.3 ADC

An apparent diffusion coefficient (ADC) is an MRI generated image that typically represents diffusion more than conventional DWI by eliminating the T2 weighting. A low *b*-value is used with other *b*-values to calculate the apparent diffusion coefficient (ADC). Tissue permeability is very well demonstrated by its ability to diffuse through cell structure. This is calculated using the apparent diffusion coefficient. This parameter is not influenced by other extrinsic and intrinsic parameters that affect conventional MR imaging, and all these calculations are done using computer software. The speciality of ADC is that it appears exactly the reverse of the diffusion-weighted imaging [79].

9.7.1.4 Time of ECHO (TE)

The time elapsed between applying one RF pulse and the maximum of the signal induced in the coil is called echo time (TE).

9.7.1.5 Diffusion-Tensor Imaging

DTI is an advanced technique that enables the precise measurement of the restricted diffusion of water in tissue and also produces images of the neural fibre tracts within the brain. DTI is an increasingly used new and advanced technique for imaging the brain white matter fibres in vivo. Diffusion tensor along with functional MRI is gaining impetus in early diagnosis. With the help of this technique, diffusion anisotropy in the tissue, the microstructure can be studied in-depth. DTI is one of the most sophisticated tools to measure water diffusion and tissue anisotropy field [1]. A symmetric unit known as the diffusion tensor accurately measures the water diffusion [80]. More than six directions can be obtained to enhance the effectiveness of the assessment of the diffusion tensor, which will dramatically boost the time taken to acquire images. Thus, two options are either increasing the number of diffusion directions or repeating the existing diffusion-weighted directions.

9.7.1.6 Fractional Anisotropy (FA)

FA value is the best DTI scalar derivative that is used to express water diffusion and the degree of anisotropy of an in vivo diffusion process that occurs in indefinite directions. These values are obtained using DTI. The diffusion-tensor data serve as the foundation for calculating eigenvectors or eigenvalues. Many parameters derived from eigenvectors are thus used for anisotropy quantification. At the moment, fractional anisotropy is the best technique for measuring diffusion anisotropy and is widely used in fibre tracking fields [81, 82].

References

1. Basser PJ, Mattiello J, LeBihan D. MR diffusion tensor spectroscopy and imaging. Biophys J. 1994;66(1):259–67. https://doi.org/10.1016/S0006-3495(94)80775-1. http://www.pubmedcentral.nih.gov/articlerender.fcgi?artid=1275686&tool=pmcentrez&rendertype=abstract.
2. Harsan LA, Poulet P, Guignard B, Steibel J, Parizel N, de Sousa PL, et al. Brain dysmyelination and recovery assessment by noninvasive in vivo diffusion tensor magnetic resonance imaging. J Neurosci Res. 2006;83(3):392–402. http://www.ncbi.nlm.nih.gov/pubmed/16397901.
3. Beaulieu C, Allen PS. Determinants of anisotropic water diffusion in nerves. Magn Reson Med. 1994;31(4):394–400. http://www.ncbi.nlm.nih.gov/pubmed/8208115.
4. Zhang J, Richards LJ, Yarowsky P, Huang H, van Zijl PCM, Mori S. Three-dimensional anatomical characterization of the developing mouse brain by diffusion tensor microimaging. Neuroimage. 2003;20(3):1639–48. http://www.ncbi.nlm.nih.gov/pubmed/14642474.
5. Mukherjee P, Miller JH, Shimony JS, Philip JV, Nehra D, Snyder AZ, et al. Diffusion-tensor MR imaging of gray and white matter development during normal human brain maturation. AJNR Am J Neuroradiol. 2002;23(9):1445–56. http://www.ncbi.nlm.nih.gov/pubmed/12372731.
6. Nieman BJ, Flenniken AM, Adamson SL, Henkelman RM, Sled JG. Anatomical phenotyping in the brain and skull of a mutant mouse by magnetic resonance imaging and computed tomography. Physiol Genomics. 2006;24(2):154–62. http://www.ncbi.nlm.nih.gov/pubmed/16410543.
7. Pagani E, Filippi M, Rocca MA, Horsfield MA. A method for obtaining tract-specific diffusion tensor MRI measurements in the presence of disease: application to patients with clinically isolated syndromes suggestive of multiple sclerosis. Neuroimage. 2005;26(1):258–65. http://www.ncbi.nlm.nih.gov/pubmed/15862226.
8. Burdette JH, Durden DD, Elster AD, Yen YF. High b-value diffusion-weighted MRI of normal brain. J Comput Assist Tomogr. 2001;25(4):515–9. http://www.ncbi.nlm.nih.gov/pubmed/11473179.
9. Chou M, Mori S. Effects of b-value and echo time on magnetic resonance diffusion tensor imaging-derived parameters at 1.5 T : a voxel-wise study. J Med Biol Eng. 2012;33(1):45–50.
10. Pierpaoli C, Jezzard P, Basser PJ, Barnett A, Di Chiro G. Diffusion tensor MR imaging of the human brain. Radiology. 1996;201(3):637–48. http://www.ncbi.nlm.nih.gov/pubmed/8939209.
11. Lee CEC, Danielian LE, Thomasson D, Baker EH. Normal regional fractional anisotropy and apparent diffusion coefficient of the brain measured on a 3 T MR scanner. Neuroradiology. 2009;51(1):3–9. http://www.ncbi.nlm.nih.gov/pubmed/18704391.
12. Huisman TAGM, Bosemani T, Poretti A. Diffusion tensor imaging for brain malformations. Neuroimaging Clin N Am. 2014;24(4):619–37. http://www.sciencedirect.com/science/article/pii/S1052514914000732.
13. Huisman TAGM, Loenneker T, Barta G, Bellemann ME, Hennig J, Fischer JE, et al. Quantitative diffusion tensor MR imaging of the brain: field strength related variance of apparent diffusion coefficient (ADC) and fractional anisotropy (FA) scalars. Eur Radiol. 2006;16(8):1651–8. http://www.ncbi.nlm.nih.gov/pubmed/16532356.
14. Snook L, Paulson L-A, Roy D, Phillips L, Beaulieu C. Diffusion tensor imaging of neurodevelopment in children and young adults. Neuroimage. 2005;26(4):1164–73. http://www.ncbi.nlm.nih.gov/pubmed/15961051.
15. van Norden AGW, de Laat KF, van Dijk EJ, van Uden IWM, van Oudheusden LJB, Gons RAR, et al. Diffusion tensor imaging and cognition in cerebral small vessel disease. Biochim Biophys Acta Mol Basis Dis. 2012;1822(3):401–7. http://www.sciencedirect.com/science/article/pii/S0925443911000913.
16. Sullivan EV, Rohlfing T, Pfefferbaum A. Longitudinal study of callosal microstructure in the normal adult aging brain using quantitative DTI fiber tracking. Dev Neuropsychol. 2010;35(3):233–56. http://www.pubmedcentral.nih.gov/articlerender.fcgi?artid=2867078&tool=pmcentrez&rendertype=abstract.

17. Hunsche S, Moseley ME, Stoeter P, Hedehus M. Diffusion-tensor MR imaging at 1.5 and 3.0 T: initial observations. Radiology. 2001;221(2):550–6. http://www.ncbi.nlm.nih.gov/pubmed/11687703.
18. Treit S, Chen Z, Rasmussen C, Beaulieu C. White matter correlates of cognitive inhibition during development: a diffusion tensor imaging study. Neuroscience. 2014;276:87–97. http://www.sciencedirect.com/science/article/pii/S030645221301035X.
19. Taylor P, Brander A, Kataja A, Saastamoinen A, Ryymin P, Huhtala H. Diffusion tensor imaging of the brain in a healthy adult population: normative values and measurement reproducibility at 3 T and 1.5 T. Acta Radiol. 2010;51(7):800–7.
20. Sexton CE, Walhovd KB, Storsve AB, Tamnes CK, Westlye LT, Johansen-Berg H, et al. Accelerated changes in white matter microstructure during aging: a longitudinal diffusion tensor imaging study. J Neurosci. 2014;34(46):15425–36. http://www.ncbi.nlm.nih.gov/pubmed/25392509.
21. Paper O. Normal development of human brain white matter from infancy to early adulthood: a diffusion tensor imaging study. Dev Neurosci. 2015;37(2):182–94.
22. Jun Q, Irvin Y, Paolo T, Yi M, Carissa S, Kang K. Tracking cerebral white matter changes across the lifespan: insights from diffusion tensor imaging studies. J Neural Transm (Vienna). 2013;120(9):1369–95.
23. Ang X, Guang-bin W, Jun-ling XU, Yong-li L, Mri C, Experimental M. Initial study of magnetic resonance diffusion tensor imaging in brain. Chin Med J. 2013;126(14):2720–4.
24. Giannelli M, Cosottini M, Michelassi MC, Lazzarotti G, Belmonte G, Bartolozzi C, et al. Dependence of brain DTI maps of fractional anisotropy and mean diffusivity on the number of diffusion weighting directions. J Appl Clin Med Phys. 2009;11(1):2927. http://www.jacmp.org/index.php/jacmp/article/view/2927/1797.
25. White matter integrity measured by fractional anisotropy correlates poorly with actual individual fiber anisotropy | Liang Zhan - Academia.edu. [cited 2014 Jun 27]. https://www.academia.edu/3512971/White_Matter_Integrity_Measured_by_Fractional_Anisotropy_Correlates_Poorly_with_Actual_Individual_Fiber_Anisotropy.
26. de Bruïne FT, van Wezel-Meijler G, Leijser LM, van den Berg-Huysmans AA, van Steenis A, van Buchem MA, et al. Tractography of developing white matter of the internal capsule and corpus callosum in very preterm infants. Eur Radiol. 2011;21(3):538–47. http://www.pubmedcentral.nih.gov/articlerender.fcgi?artid=3032189&tool=pmcentrez&rendertype=abstract.
27. Chang MC, Jang SH. Corpus callosum injury in patients with diffuse axonal injury: a diffusion tensor imaging study. NeuroRehabilitation. 2010;26(4):339–45. http://www.ncbi.nlm.nih.gov/pubmed/20555157.
28. Liu F, Vidarsson L, Winter JD, Tran H, Kassner A. Sex differences in the human corpus callosum microstructure: a combined T2 myelin-water and diffusion tensor magnetic resonance imaging study. Brain Res. 2010;1343:37–45. http://www.ncbi.nlm.nih.gov/pubmed/20435024.
29. Provenzale JM, Isaacson J, Chen S, Stinnett S, Liu C. Correlation of apparent diffusion coefficient and fractional anisotropy values in the developing infant brain. AJR Am J Roentgenol. 2010;195(6):W456–62. http://www.pubmedcentral.nih.gov/articlerender.fcgi?artid=3640803&tool=pmcentrez&rendertype=abstract.
30. Kim EY, Park H-J, Kim D-H, Lee S-K, Kim J. Measuring fractional anisotropy of the corpus callosum using diffusion tensor imaging: mid-sagittal versus axial imaging planes. Korean J Radiol. 2008;9(5):391–5. http://www.pubmedcentral.nih.gov/articlerender.fcgi?artid=2627217&tool=pmcentrez&rendertype=abstract
31. Rutgers DR, Fillard P, Paradot G, Tadié M, Lasjaunias P, Ducreux D. Diffusion tensor imaging characteristics of the corpus callosum in mild, moderate, and severe traumatic brain injury. AJNR Am J Neuroradiol. 2008;29(9):1730–5. http://www.ncbi.nlm.nih.gov/pubmed/18617586.
32. Hasan KM, Gupta RK, Santos RM, Wolinsky JS, Narayana PA. Diffusion tensor fractional anisotropy of the normal-appearing seven segments of the corpus callosum in healthy adults and relapsing-remitting multiple sclerosis patients. J Magn Reson Imaging. 2005;21(6):735–43. http://www.ncbi.nlm.nih.gov/pubmed/15906348.

33. Jeong HK, Lee S-K, Kim DI, Heo JH. The usefulness of fractional anisotropy maps in localization of lacunar infarctions in striatum, internal capsule and thalamus. Neuroradiology. 2005;47(4):267–70. http://www.ncbi.nlm.nih.gov/pubmed/15806429.
34. Hakulinen U, Brander A, Ryymin P, Öhman J, Soimakallio S, Helminen M, et al. Repeatability and variation of region-of-interest methods using quantitative diffusion tensor MR imaging of the brain. BMC Med Imaging. 2012;12:30. http://www.pubmedcentral.nih.gov/articlerender.fcgi?artid=3533516&tool=pmcentrez&rendertype=abstract.
35. Fox RJ, Sakaie K, Lee J-C, Debbins JP, Liu Y, Arnold DL, et al. A validation study of multicenter diffusion tensor imaging: reliability of fractional anisotropy and diffusivity values. AJNR Am J Neuroradiol. 2012;33(4):695–700. http://www.ncbi.nlm.nih.gov/pubmed/22173748.
36. Murphy ML, Frodl T. Meta-analysis of diffusion tensor imaging studies shows altered fractional anisotropy occurring in distinct brain areas in association with depression. Biol Mood Anxiety Disord. 2011;1(1):3. http://www.biolmoodanxietydisord.com/content/1/1/3.
37. Brander A, Kataja A, Saastamoinen A, Ryymin P, Huhtala H, Ohman J, et al. Diffusion tensor imaging of the brain in a healthy adult population: normative values and measurement reproducibility at 3 T and 1.5 T. Acta Radiol. 2010;51(7):800–7. http://informahealthcare.com/doi/abs/10.3109/02841851.2010.495351.
38. Giannelli M, Cosottini M, Michelassi MC, Lazzarotti G, Belmonte G, Bartolozzi C, et al. Dependence of brain DTI maps of fractional anisotropy and mean diffusivity on the number of diffusion weighting directions. J Appl Clin Med Phys. 2009;11(1):2927. http://www.ncbi.nlm.nih.gov/pubmed/20160677.
39. Bisdas S, Bohning DEE, Besenski N, Nicholas JSS, Rumboldt Z. Reproducibility, interrater agreement, and age-related changes of fractional anisotropy measures at 3T in healthy subjects: effect of the applied b-value. AJNR Am J Neuroradiol. 2008;29(6):1128–33. http://www.ajnr.org/cgi/doi/10.3174/ajnr.A1044.
40. Mandl CW, Schnack HG, Zwiers MP, Van Der SA. Functional diffusion tensor imaging: measuring task- related fractional anisotropy changes in the human brain along white matter tracts. PLoS One. 2008;3(11):e3631.
41. Schlu M, Drescher R, Rexilius J, Lukas C, Hahn HK, Przuntek H, et al. Diffusion tensor imaging-based fractional anisotropy quantification in the corticospinal tract of patients with amyotrophic lateral sclerosis using a probabilistic mixture model. AJNR Am J Neuroradiol. 2007;28(4):724–30.
42. Farrell JAD, Landman BA, Jones CK, Smith SA, Prince JL, van Zijl PCM, et al. Effects of signal-to-noise ratio on the accuracy and reproducibility of diffusion tensor imaging-derived fractional anisotropy, mean diffusivity, and principal eigenvector measurements at 1.5 T. J Magn Reson Imaging. 2007;26(3):756–67. http://www.pubmedcentral.nih.gov/articlerender.fcgi?artid=2862967&tool=pmcentrez&rendertype=abstract.
43. Löbel U, Sedlacik J, Güllmar D, Kaiser WA, Reichenbach JR, Mentzel H. Diffusion tensor imaging: the normal evolution of ADC, RA, FA, and eigenvalues studied in multiple anatomical regions of the brain. Neuroradiology. 2009;51(4):253–63. http://media.proquest.com/media/pq/classic/doc/1664748221/fmt/pi/rep/NONE?hl=&cit:auth=Löbel,+Ulrike;Sedlacik,+Jan;Güllmar,+Daniel;Kaiser,+Werner+A;Reichenbach,+Jürgen+R;Mentzel,+Hans-joachim&cit:title=Diffusion+te.
44. Mole JP, Subramanian L, Bracht T, Morris H, Metzler-Baddeley C, Linden DEJ. Increased fractional anisotropy in the motor tracts of Parkinson's disease suggests compensatory neuroplasticity or selective neurodegeneration. Eur Radiol. 2016;26(10):3327–35.
45. Ibarretxe-Bilbao N, Junque C, Marti MJ, Valldeoriola F, Vendrell P, Bargallo N, et al. Olfactory impairment in Parkinson's disease and white matter abnormalities in central olfactory areas: a voxel-based diffusion tensor imaging study. Mov Disord. 2010;25(12):1888–94.
46. Georgiopoulos C, Warntjes M, Dizdar N, Zachrisson H, Engström M, Haller S, et al. Olfactory impairment in Parkinson's disease studied with diffusion tensor and magnetization transfer imaging. J Parkinsons Dis. 2017;7(2):301–11.

47. Joshi N, Rolheiser TM, Fisk JD, McKelvey JR, Schoffer K, Phillips G, et al. Lateralized microstructural changes in early-stage Parkinson's disease in anterior olfactory structures, but not in substantia nigra. J Neurol. 2017;264(7):1497–505.
48. Rolheiser TM, Fulton HG, Good KP, Fisk JD, McKelvey JR, Scherfler C, et al. Diffusion tensor imaging and olfactory identification testing in early-stage Parkinson's disease. J Neurol. 2011;258(7):1254–60.
49. Kim M, Park H. Using tractography to distinguish SWEDD from Parkinson's disease patients based on connectivity. Parkinsons Dis. 2016;2016:8704910.
50. Cousineau M, Jodoin PM, Morency FC, Rozanski V, Grand'Maison M, Bedell BJ, et al. A test-retest study on Parkinson's PPMI dataset yields statistically significant white matter fascicles. NeuroImage Clin. 2017;16:222–33.
51. Zhang K, Yu C, Zhang Y, Wu X, Zhu C. Voxel-based analysis of diffusion tensor indices in the brain in patients with Parkinson's disease. Eur J Radiol. 2017;77(2):269–73. https://doi.org/10.1016/j.ejrad.2009.07.032.
52. Zhan W, Kang GA, Glass GA, Zhang Y, Shirley C, Millin R, et al. Regional alterations of brain microstructure in Parkinson's disease using diffusion tensor imaging. Mov Disord. 2012;27(1):90–7.
53. Langley J, Huddleston DE, Merritt M, Chen X, McMurray R, Silver M, et al. Diffusion tensor imaging of the substantia nigra in Parkinson's disease revisited. Hum Brain Mapp. 2016;37(7):2547–56.
54. Duncan GW, Firbank MJ, Yarnall AJ, Khoo TK, Brooks DJ, Barker RA, et al. Gray and white matter imaging: a biomarker for cognitive impairment in early Parkinson's disease? Mov Disord. 2016;31(1):103–10.
55. Chen N-K, Chou Y, Sundman M, Hickey P, Kasoff WS, Bernstein A, et al. Alteration of diffusion-tensor MRI measures in brain regions involved in early stages of Parkinson's disease. Brain Connect. 2018;8(6):343–9. http://www.liebertpub.com/doi/10.1089/brain.2017.0558.
56. Gattellaro G, Minati L, Grisoli M, Mariani C, Carella F, Osio M, et al. White matter involvement in idiopathic Parkinson disease: a diffusion tensor imaging study. AJNR Am J Neuroradiol. 2009;30(6):1222–6.
57. Zhang Y, Schuff N, Jahng G-H, Bayne W, Mori S, Schad L, et al. Diffusion tensor imaging of cingulum fibers in mild cognitive impairment and Alzheimer disease. Neurology. 2007;68(1):13–9. http://www.pubmedcentral.nih.gov/articlerender.fcgi?artid=1941719&tool=pmcentrez&rendertype=abstract.
58. Cochrane CJ. Diffusion tensor imaging in parkinsonian syndromes: a systematic review and meta-analysis. Neurology. 2013;80(9):857–64.
59. Schwarz ST, Abaei M, Gontu V, Morgan PS, Bajaj N, Auer DP. Diffusion tensor imaging of nigral degeneration in Parkinson's disease: a region-of-interest and voxel-based study at 3 T and systematic review with meta-analysis. NeuroImage Clin. 2013;3:481–8. https://doi.org/10.1016/j.nicl.2013.10.006.
60. Atkinson-Clement C, Pinto S, Eusebio A, Coulon O. Diffusion tensor imaging in Parkinson's disease: review and meta-analysis. NeuroImage Clin. 2017;16:98–110. https://doi.org/10.1016/j.nicl.2017.07.011.
61. Cochrane CJ, Ebmeier KP. Diffusion tensor imaging in parkinsonian syndromes: a systematic review and meta-analysis. Neurology. 2013;80(9):857–64.
62. Wen MC, Heng HSE, Ng SYE, Tan LCS, Chan LL, Tan EK. White matter microstructural characteristics in newly diagnosed Parkinson's disease: an unbiased whole-brain study. Sci Rep. 2016;6:35601. https://doi.org/10.1038/srep35601.
63. Farrell JA, Landman BA, Jones CK, Smith SA, Prince JL, Van ZPC, et al. Effects of diffusion weighting scheme and SNR on DTI-derived fractional anisotropy at 1.5T Introduction. Proc Intl Soc Mag Reson Med. 2006;993:2000.
64. Smith SM, Johansen-Berg H, Jenkinson M, Rueckert D, Nichols TE, Klein JC, et al. Acquisition and voxelwise analysis of multi-subject diffusion data with tract-based spatial statistics. Nat Protoc. 2007;2(3):499–503.

65. Concha L, Bouchard T, Wiltshire K, Concha L, Gee M, Bouchard T. Corpus callosum and cingulum tractography in Parkinson's disease. Can J Neurol Sci. 2010;37(5):595–600.
66. Nilsson M, Eriksson B, Surova Y, Szczepankiewicz F, La J, Leemans A, et al. Assessment of global and regional diffusion changes along white matter tracts in Parkinsonian disorders by MR tractography. PLoS One. 2013;8(6):e66022.
67. Keller J, Rulseh AM, Komárek A, Latnerová I, Rusina R, Brožová H, et al. New non-linear color look-up table for visualization of brain fractional anisotropy based on normative measurements—principals and first clinical use. PLoS One. 2013;8(8):1–7. http://www.ncbi.nlm.nih.gov/pubmed/23990954.
68. Aquino D, Contarino V, Albanese A, Minati L, Farina L, Grisoli M, et al. Substantia nigra in Parkinson's disease: a multimodal MRI comparison between early and advanced stages of the disease. Neurol Sci. 2014;35(5):753–8.
69. Report S. Early pathological changes in the parkinsonian brain demonstrated by diffusion tensor MRI. J Neurol Neurosurg Psychiatry. 2004;75(3):481–4.
70. Mormina E, Arrigo A, Calamuneri A, Granata F, Quartarone A, Ghilardi MF, et al. Diffusion tensor imaging parameters' changes of cerebellar hemispheres in Parkinson's disease. Neuroradiology. 2015;57(3):327–34.
71. Lu C, Ng S, Weng Y, Cheng J. Alterations of diffusion tensor MRI parameters in the brains of patients with Parkinson's disease compared with normal brains: possible diagnostic use. Eur Radiol. 2016;26(11):3978–88. https://doi.org/10.1007/s00330-016-4232-7.
72. Auning E, Kjærvik VK, Selnes P, Aarsland D, Haram A, Bjørnerud A, et al. White matter integrity and cognition in Parkinson's disease: a cross-sectional study. BMJ Open. 2014;4(1):e003976.
73. Lenfeldt N, Hansson W, Larsson A, Nyberg L, Birgander R, Forsgren L. Diffusion tensor imaging and correlations to Parkinson rating scales. J Neurol. 2013;260(11):2823–30. http://www.ncbi.nlm.nih.gov/pubmed/23974647.
74. Meijer FJA, Van Rumund A, Tuladhar AM. Conventional 3T brain MRI and diffusion tensor imaging in the diagnostic workup of early stage parkinsonism. Neuroradiology. 2015;57(7):655–69. https://doi.org/10.1007/s00234-015-1515-7.
75. Saotome K, Ishimori Y, Isobe T, Satou E. [Comparison of diffusion tensor imaging-derived fractional anisotropy in multiple centers for identical human subjects]. Nihon Hoshasen Gijutsu Gakkai Zasshi. 2012;68(9):1242–9.
76. Fick's insight on liquid diffusion. [cited 2014 Jul 16]. http://www.olemiss.edu/sciencenet/saltnet/fick_insights_EOS.pdf.
77. Beluffi G. Diffusion-weighted MR imaging. Applications in the body D.M. Koh H.C. Thoeni (Eds.). Radiol Med. 2011;116(3):499–500. http://link.springer.com/10.1007/s11547-011-0638-z.
78. Bammer R, Holdsworth SJ, Veldhuis WB, Skare ST. New methods in diffusion-weighted and diffusion tensor imaging. Magn Reson Imaging Clin N Am. 2009;17(2):175–204. http://www.pubmedcentral.nih.gov/articlerender.fcgi?artid=2768271&tool=pmcentrez&rendertype=abstract.
79. Neil JJ. Diffusion imaging concepts for clinicians. J Magn Reson Imaging. 2008;27(1):1–7. http://www.ncbi.nlm.nih.gov/pubmed/18050325.
80. Basser PJ, Jones DK. Diffusion-tensor MRI: theory, experimental design and data analysis—a technical review. NMR Biomed. 2002;15(7–8):456–67. http://www.ncbi.nlm.nih.gov/pubmed/12489095.
81. Pierpaoli C, Basser PJ. Toward a quantitative assessment of diffusion anisotropy. Magn Reson Med. 1996;36(6):893–906. http://www.ncbi.nlm.nih.gov/pubmed/8946355.
82. Yoshiura T, Wu O, Zaheer A, Reese TG, Sorensen AG. Highly diffusion-sensitized MRI of brain: dissociation of gray and white matter. Magn Reson Med. 2001;45(5):734–40. http://www.ncbi.nlm.nih.gov/pubmed/11323798.

FA Characteristics as Imaging Biomarkers Among the Indian Population in Early Parkinson's Disease

10

10.1 Background

The previous chapter outlined the clinical evidence for FA in PD. In this chapter, we will discuss important imaging biomarker findings of FA in early PD with an emphasis on key findings in the Indian population. There is a lack of data for the Indian population on FA characteristics as imaging biomarkers in early PD.

PD is a dopamine-specific dysfunction characterized by one or more motor system-related symptoms such as slowness of movement, rest involuntary movements, high stiffness and postural instability. Because the onset of PD in the brain is a relatively slow process, basic MRI scans fail to detect any abnormalities associated with it. The primary function of MRI has been to depict atrophy changes, but its overall diagnostic significance is low. Early detection of PD will eventually improve the overall quality of life and reduce morbidity in PD patients through prompt medication and therapy.

The search and need for an imaging biomarker in PD are critical, and it will have a substantial effect on the patient's future. DTI has begun to show promising results in assessing GM and WM abnormalities, which may serve as an imaging marker for the progression of PD. FA is the preferred and most robust quantitative measure of diffusion among the DTI scalar derivatives for clinical interpretation.

The literature still lacks information beyond the SN and a few cortical and subcortical GM regions of the brain for PD. As a result, the development of specific imaging biomarkers for early PD diagnosis will significantly benefit PD patients and their diagnosis and management.

A case-control prospective study design will be discussed to better understand imaging biomarkers and FA in early PD. We used data from 80 Indians (40 controls + 40 cases) from Kasturba Hospital in Manipal, Karnataka, India, to better understand FA characteristics as an imaging biomarker in early PD in the Indian

R. P. Kotian, P. Koteshwar, *Diffusion Tensor Imaging and Fractional Anisotropy*,
https://doi.org/10.1007/978-981-19-5001-8_10

population. The role of DTI in both the GM and WM brain areas was investigated in early PD cases and controls using FA with the fixed region of interest (ROI) techniques.

10.2 Clinical and Demographic Characteristics

After preliminary screening, healthy participants with no neurological dysfunction were recruited for the control group. The current study included 65 healthy participants with no neurological problems in the control group and 65 early PD patients with a disease history of 6 months to 3 years.

Patients with early PD who were clinically proven to have PD using UPDRS test score results were included. The UPDRS score was also useful in categorizing and describing the severity of PD patients. In the current study, the following inclusion and exclusion criteria were used to recruit participants in both groups. Figures 10.1, 10.2, 10.3, 10.4, 10.5 and 10.6 depict the GM and WM regions of the brain used to investigate FA characteristics.

Inclusion Criteria

- Participants who do not have any neurological dysfunction
- Participants with clinically diagnosed early PD (0–3 years). Subjects meeting the requirements for idiopathic PD (UK Parkinson's Disease Society Brain Bank)
- Subjects' age range: 40–75 years

Exclusion Criteria

- Participants were found to have structural neurological problems and lesions on a standard MR imaging.
- Participants categorically contraindicated to MR imaging.
- Participants with vascular parkinsonism, MSA with PD and dementia-related PD with Lewy bodies were excluded from the study. Table 10.1 depicts the demographic and clinical information from the current study.

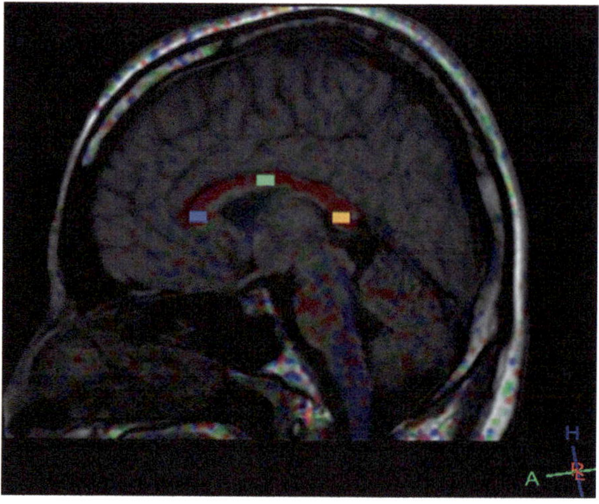

Fig. 10.1 FA value extraction at CC (genu, body and splenium)

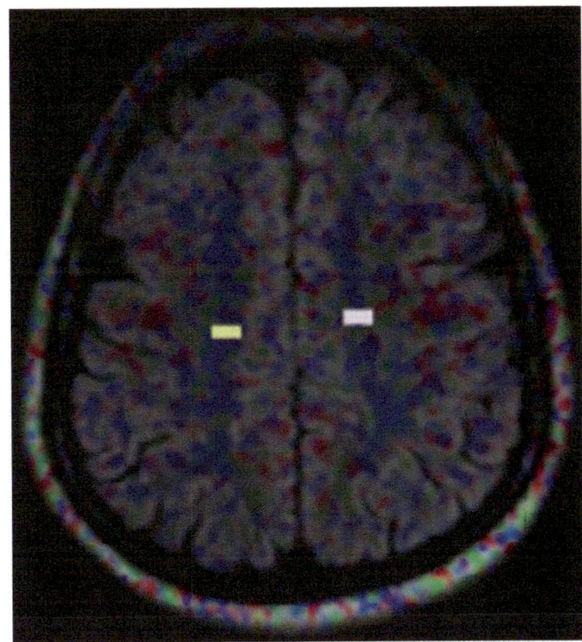

Fig. 10.2 FA value extraction at CS

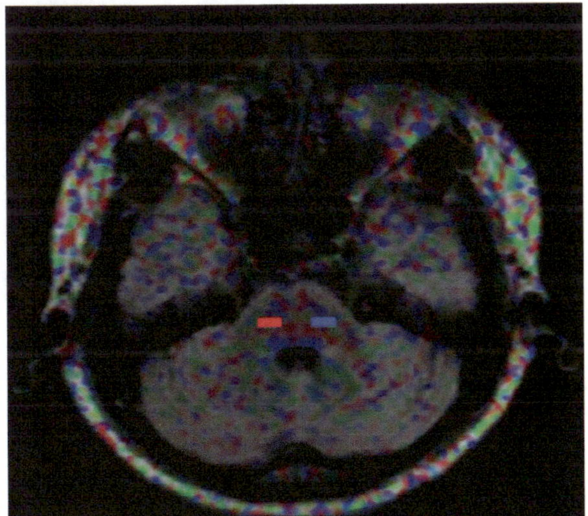

Fig. 10.3 FA value extraction at pons

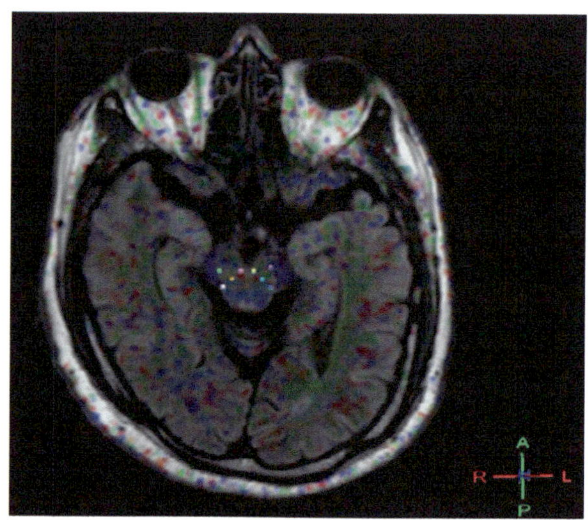

Fig. 10.4 *FA value extraction* at SN and cerebral peduncles

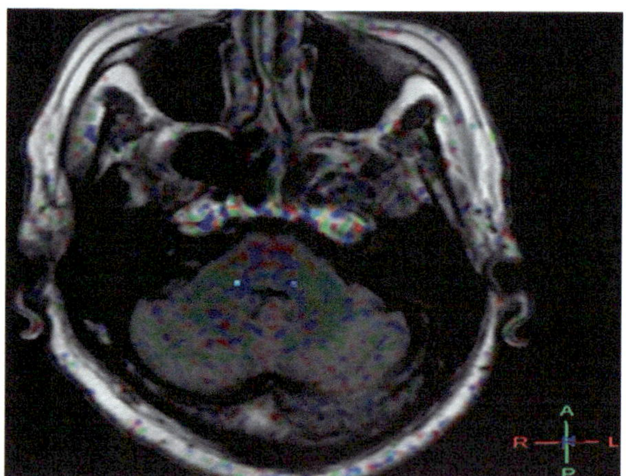

Fig. 10.5 *FA value extraction* at cerebellar peduncles

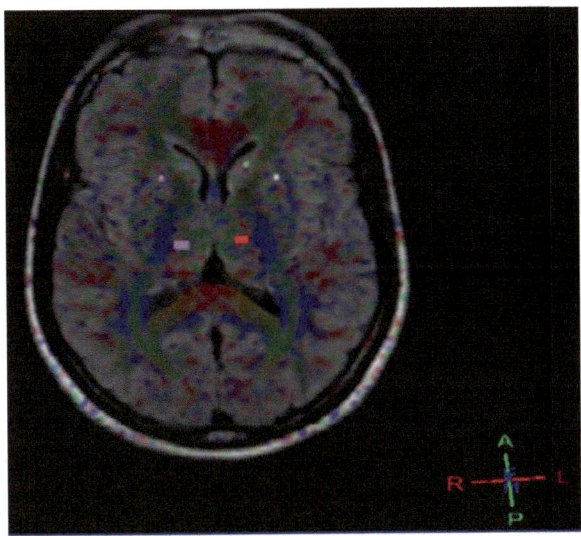

Fig. 10.6 *FA value extraction* at CN, putamen and thalamus

Table 10.1 Demographic and clinical information

$N = 40$	PD	Controls	p-Value
Age (Y)[a]	63.25 ± 6.49[a]	64.06 ± 7.38[a]	0.435[c]
Sex (M/F)[b]	40:25[b]	40:25[b]	0.386[c]
Disease duration (MT)[b]	11 ± 2.25[b]	NA	NA

[a]The age and PD duration are reported as Mean ± standard deviation
[b]*Y* years, *M* males, *F* females, *MT* months
[c]No statistical variation ($p > 0.05$) between the two groups, *NA* not applicable

10.2.1 UPDRS Criteria in PD

10.2.1.1 Step 1: Parkinsonian Syndrome Diagnosis

- Bradykinesia
- At least one of the following:
  - Muscular rigidity
  - 4–6 Hz rest tremor
  - Postural instability not caused by primary visual, vestibular, cerebellar or proprioceptive dysfunction

10.2.1.2 Step 2: Exclusion Criteria for Parkinson's Disease

- History of repeated strokes with the stepwise progression of parkinsonian features
- History of repeated head injury
- History of definite encephalitis
- Oculogyric crises

- Neuroleptic treatment at the onset of symptoms
- More than one affected relative
- Sustained remission
- Strictly unilateral features after 3 years
- Supranuclear gaze palsy
- Cerebellar signs
- Early severe autonomic involvement
- Early severe dementia with disturbances of memory, language and praxis
- Babinski sign
- Presence of cerebral tumor or communication hydrocephalus on an imaging study
- A negative response to large doses of levodopa in the absence of malabsorption
- MPTP exposure

10.2.1.3 Step 3: Supportive Prospective Positive Criteria for Parkinson's Disease [1]

Three or more are required for the diagnosis of definite Parkinson's disease in combination with step 1:

- Unilateral onset
- Rest tremor present
- Progressive disorder
- Persistent asymmetry affecting side of onset most
- Excellent response (70–100%) to levodopa
- Severe levodopa-induced chorea
- Levodopa response for 5 years or more
- The clinical course of 10 years or more [1]

10.2.2 Predictive Performance of Diffusion-Tensor Imaging

The study's findings reported FA at different GM and WM regions of the brain which are detailed in Table 10.2. In the PD group, we observed the highest FA of 0.713 at the splenium of the CC and the lowest FA of 0.410 at the caudate nucleus. Similarly, the control group reported the highest FA of 0.694 at the splenium of the CC and the lowest FA of 0.453 at the CN. The FA values were reported using a *b*-value of 1000 s/mm^2 and a TE of 100 (ms) as a fixed protocol in both the PD and control groups as depicted in Table 10.2.

Table 10.2 Mean and SD: FA in PD vs. control group

Brain areas	(Control) FA (mean ± standard deviation)	(PD) FA (mean ± standard deviation)
CC (genu)	0.558 ± 0.06	0.659 ± 0.07
CC (body)	0.564 ± 0.11	0.627 ± 0.11
CC (splenium)	0.694 ± 0.13	0.713 ± 0.06
CS	0.530 ± 0.06	0.556 ± 0.06
Pons	0.585 ± 0.04	0.609 ± 0.05
CN	0.453 ± 0.14	0.410 ± 0.09
Putamen	0.531 ± 0.07	0.470 ± 0.08
Thalamus	0.509 ± 0.07	0.513 ± 0.08
SN	0.608 ± 0.07	0.423 ± 0.01
Cerebral peduncles	0.613 ± 0.05	0.646 ± 0.11
Cerebellar peduncles	0.509 ± 0.11	0.566 ± 0.09

10.3 Imaging Biomarkers in Early PD

Sir James Parkinson, a marvelous scientist, gave us an insight into PD in 1817, which was later refined by Jean-Martin Charcot in the late nineteenth century to include atypical parkinsonian types known as Parkinson-Plus syndrome. PD is currently the second most common neurodegenerative disease, with an estimated ten million cases worldwide [2]. Years of scientific data analysis and investigations have resulted in a lack of clarity on imaging markers for the early detection of PD using diagnostic medical imaging techniques. In the following section of this chapter, we will go over some of the most important findings from the current study on imaging markers and early PD. Figures 10.1, 10.2, 10.3, 10.4, 10.5 and 10.6 show the ROI methods used in the study to obtain FA values in the GM and WM of the brain.

10.3.1 Independent Sample *t*-Test Findings Among Indian Population

The statistical analysis to determine the relevance of FA in the control and PD groups is depicted in Table 10.3. There was a statistically significant difference between the PD and control groups in the following brain regions: CC (genu and body), SN, putamen, SN, cerebral peduncles and pons. The use of ROC analysis was initiated to further evaluate positive predictors.

10.3.2 Brain Region-Specific FA Range

This study also reported the FA range in WM and GM regions of the brain as depicted in Table 10.4. A range of FA would always be beneficial while dealing with

Table 10.3 Independent t-test findings: PD vs. control group

Brain areas	p-Value
Genu of CC	0.000*
Body of CC	0.014*
Splenium of CC	0.757
CS	0.083
PO	0.034*
CN	0.163
P	0.000*
T	0.214
SN	0.000*
CP	0.003*
CPP	0.411

*Statistically significant values; *CC* corpus callosum, *CS* centrum semiovale, *CP* cerebral peduncles, *CN* caudate nucleus, *CPP* cerebellar peduncles, *P* putamen, *PO* pons, *SN* substantia nigra, *T* thalamus

Table 10.4 FA value range at WM and GM brain areas

Brain areas	FA range (control)	FA range (PD)
CC (genu)	0.510–0.780	0.343–0.742
CC (body)	0.446–0.811	0.420–0.817
CC (splenium)	0.56–0.860	0.550–0.791
CS	0.404–0.638	0.416–0.71
PO	0.525–0.681	0.553–0.715
CN	0.278–0.753	0.274–0.694
P	0.371–0.710	0.260–0.672
T	0.341–0.606	0.420–0.585
SN	0.470–0.717	0.394–0.437
CP	0.411–0.847	0.380–0.767
CPP	0.227–0.693	0.421–0.732

CC corpus callosum, *CS* centrum semiovale, *CP* cerebral peduncles, *CN* caudate nucleus, *CPP* cerebellar peduncles, *P* putamen, *PO* pons, *SN* substantia nigra, *T* thalamus

a broad spectrum of PD patients whose disease duration may vary from 12 months to 36 months. This FA range can be used to categorize PD into early- and late-stage categories. The range of FA values using b-value, 1000 s/mm^2, and TE, 100 ms, as a combination has been reported in both PD and control groups in the study findings.

10.3.3 Receiver Operator Characteristics Curve Findings in Early PD

To further add insight on imaging markers, curve ROC analysis was performed for the GM and WM brain areas which were earlier found statistically relevant using the independent sample t-test. A summary of the results obtained using ROC

Table 10.5 ROC analysis for positive predictors

Predictors	Curve area	Cut-off	Sensitivity	Specificity
CC (genu)	0.835	0.6074	0.8	0.85
CC (body)	0.687	0.5544	0.8	0.625
PO	0.631	0.586	0.575	0.475
P	0.742	0.499	0.0750	0.725
SN	1.0	0.484	1.000	1.000
CP	0.740	0.718	0.75	0.70

CC corpus callosum, *CS* centrum semiovale, *CP* cerebral peduncles, *CN* caudate nucleus, *P* putamen, *PO* pons, *SN* substantia nigra

analysis is depicted in Table 10.5. The ROC analysis was mainly performed to find the specificity and sensitivity of the regions of the brain GM and WM which were statistically significant using an independent sample *t*-test. Our study findings reported good sensitivity and specificity for all regions of the brain in the study except pons. Substantia nigra showed a sensitivity and specificity of 100% in identifying early PD cases from healthy controls. A detailed explanation of results obtained from ROC analysis is described below:

Corpus callosum

(a) The ROC analysis for FA in the genu of the CC showed an AUC of 0.836 ± 0.04. The reported values were between 0.741 and 0.932 (95% CI). As shown in Fig. 10.7, the determined optimal cut-off point was 0.6075 with a sensitivity of 0.8 and a specificity of 0.85 for the PD patients.
(b) The ROC analysis for the FA in the body of the CC showed an AUC of 0.688 ± 0.06. The reported values were between 0.564 and 0.812 (95% CI). As shown in Fig. 10.8, the determined optimal cut-off point was 0.554 with a sensitivity of 0.8 and a specificity of 0.625 for the PD patients.

Pons

(c) The ROC analysis for the FA in the pons showed an AUC of 0.630 ± 0.06. The reported values were between 0.508 and 0.752 (95% CI). As shown in Fig. 10.9, the determined optimal cut-off point was 0.586 with a sensitivity of 0.575 and a specificity of 0.475 for the PD patients.

Putamen

(d) The ROC analysis for the FA in the putamen showed an AUC of 0.74 1 ± 0.05. The reported values were between 0.626 and0.857 (95% CI). As shown in Fig. 10.10, the determined optimal cut-off point was 0.498 with a sensitivity of 0.75 and a specificity of 0.725 for the PD patients.

Substantia Nigra

(e) The ROC analysis for the FA in the substantia nigra showed an AUC of 1. The reported values were between 1.00 and 1.00 (95% CI). As shown in Fig. 10.11, the determined optimal cut-off point was 0.484 with a sensitivity of 100% and a specificity of 100% for the PD patients.

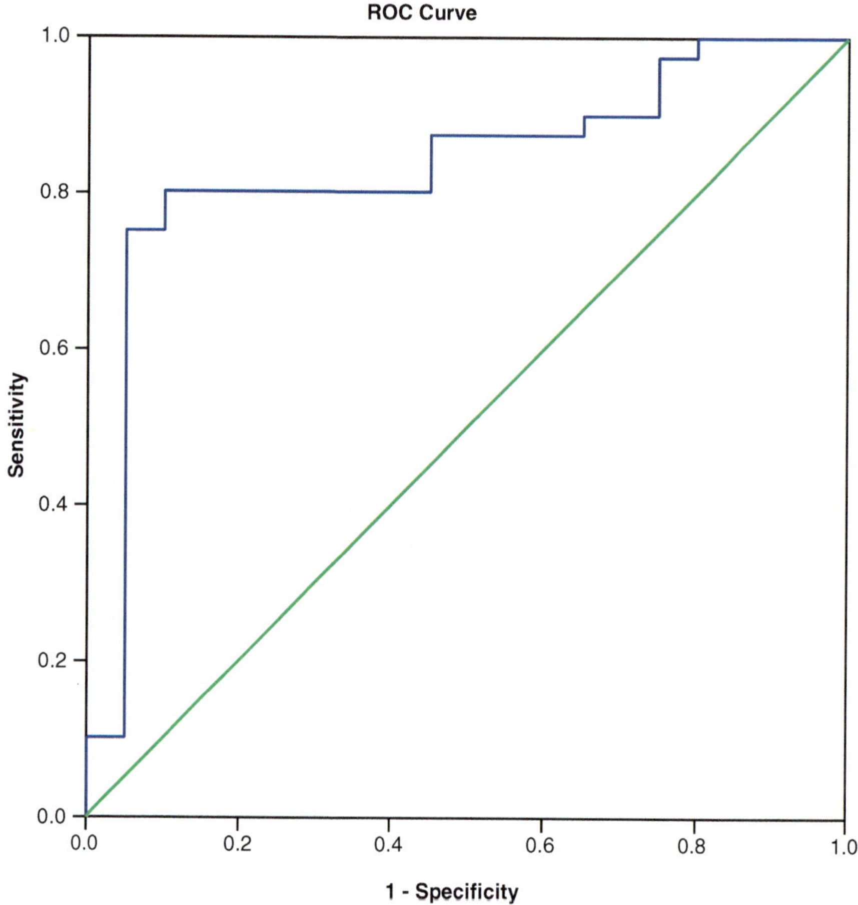

Fig. 10.7 ROC at the genu of CC. **The AUC is a measure of performance for comparison between controls and PD patients*

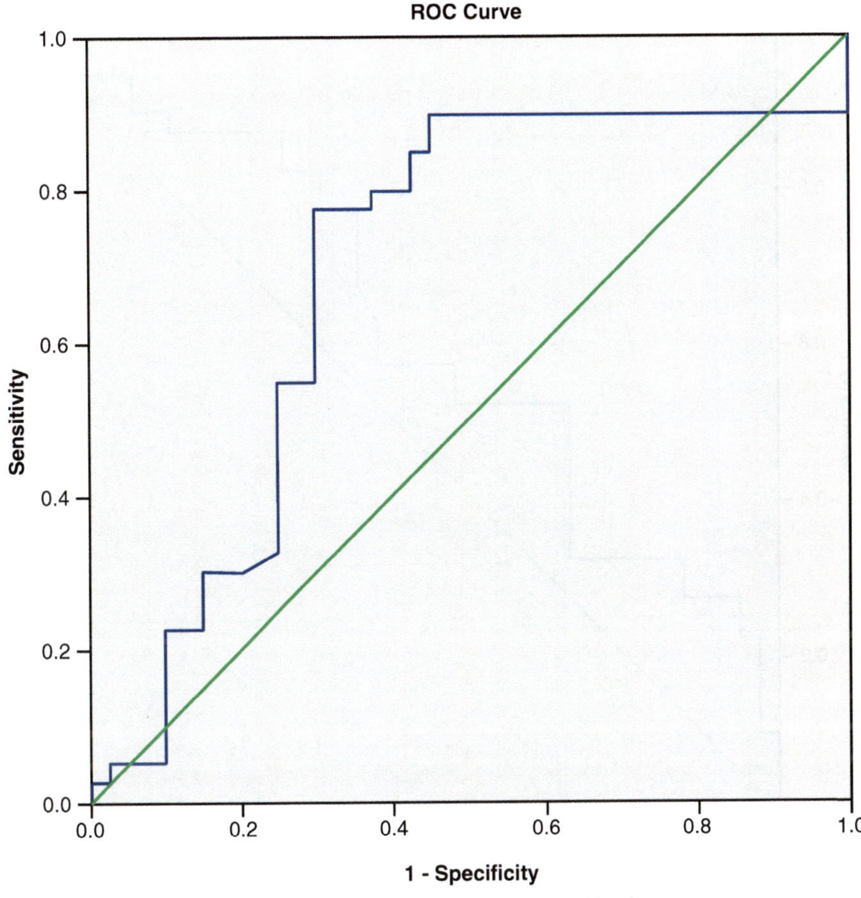

Fig. 10.8 ROC at the body of CC

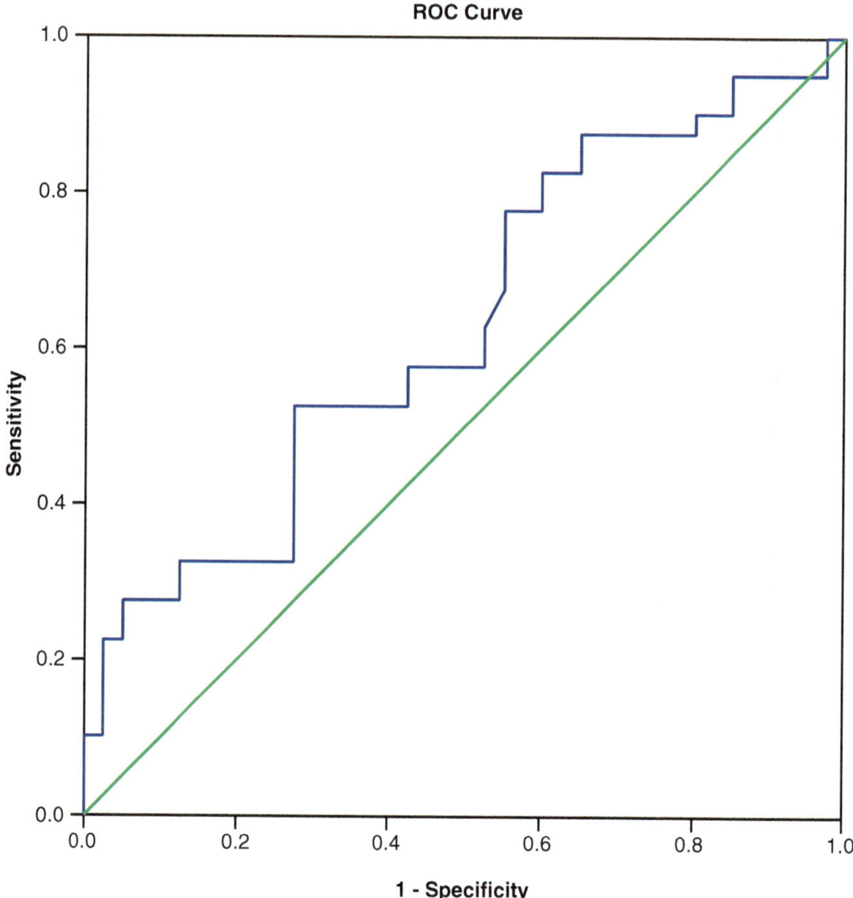

Fig. 10.9 ROC at the pons

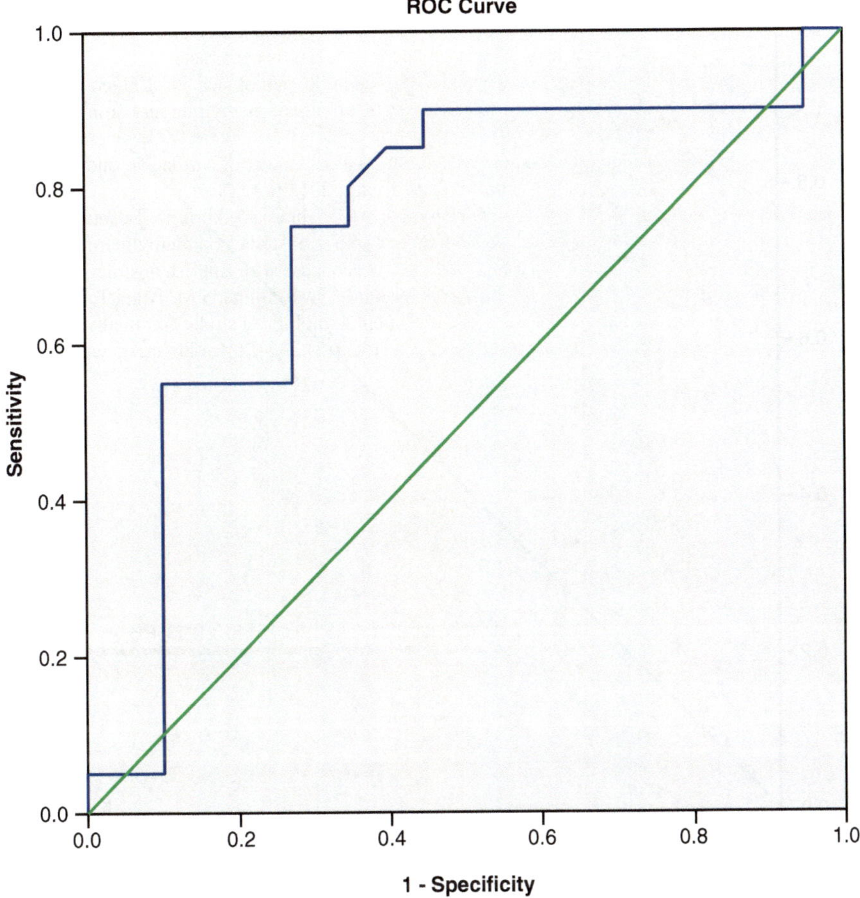

Fig. 10.10 ROC at the putamen

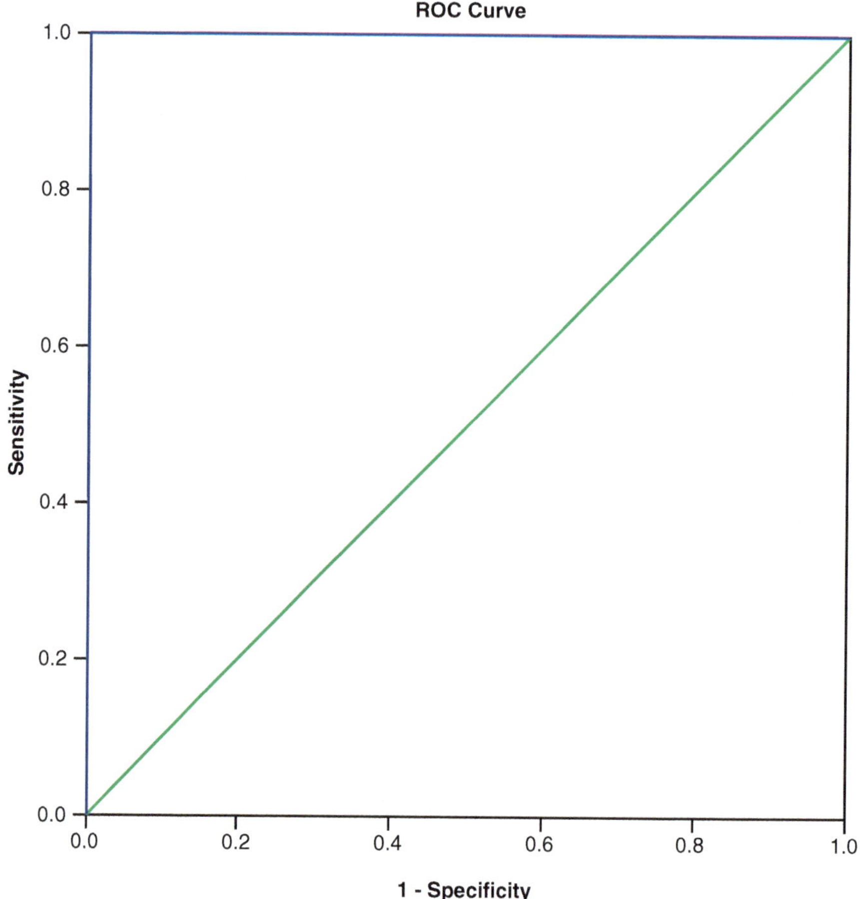

Fig. 10.11 ROC at the SN

Cerebral Peduncles

(f) The ROC analysis for the FA in the cerebral peduncles showed an AUC of 0.741 ± 0.05. The reported values were between 0.628 and 0.855. As shown in Fig. 10.12, the determined optimal cut-off point was 0.719 with a sensitivity of 0.8 and a specificity of 0.85 for the PD patients.

10.3.4 Significant Predictors for PD vs. Control Group

Figure 10.13 depicts a comparison of FA in the significant predicting brain areas between the control and PD groups. Finally, the study found a statistically relevant difference between the PD and control groups in the CC (genu and body), SN, putamen and cerebral peduncles. Pons was found to be insignificant as a predictor. The putamen, CC and cerebral peduncles were found to be the best predictors of early PD.

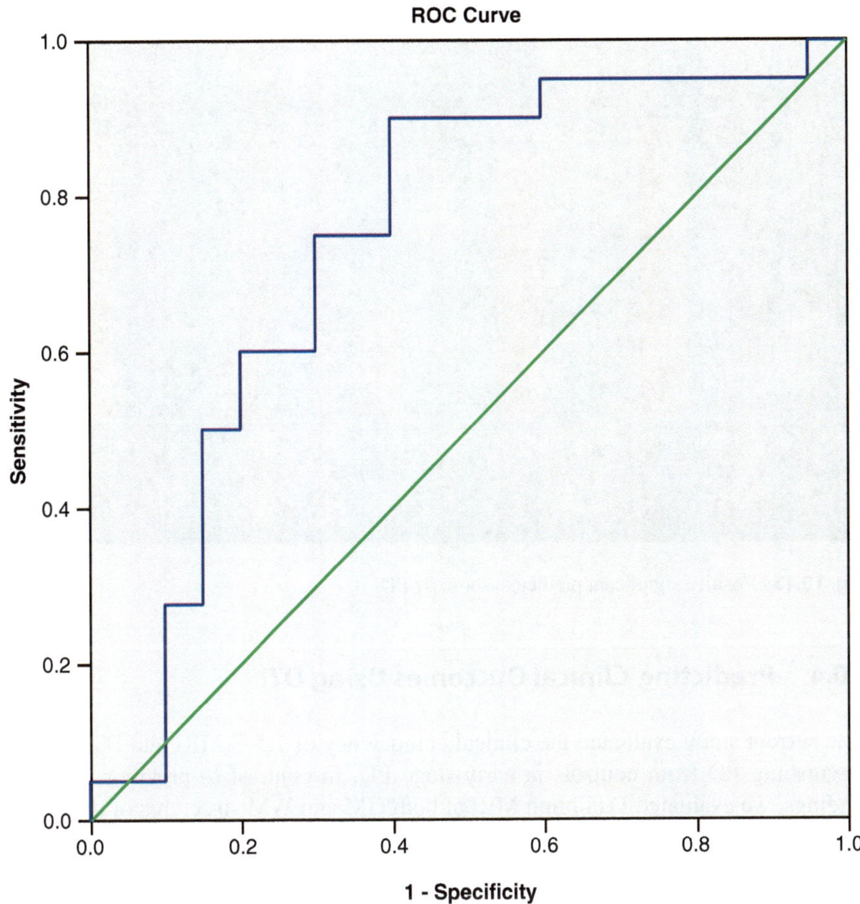

Fig. 10.12 ROC at the cerebral peduncles

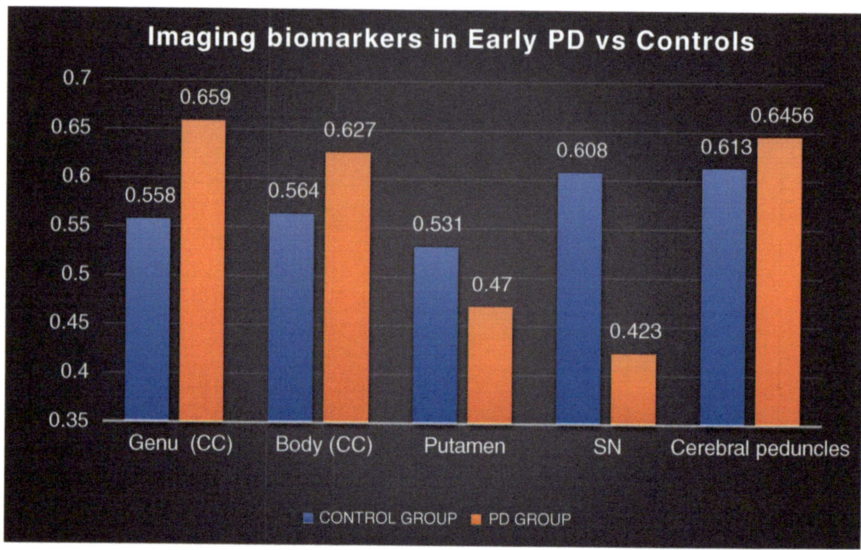

Fig. 10.13 Positive significant predictors for early PD

10.4 Predicting Clinical Outcomes Using DTI

The current study evaluated the clinical competency of 1.5-T MRI and DTI in distinguishing PD from controls in early-stage PD. In contrast to previous research findings, we evaluated DTI brain MRI at both GM and WM structures of the brain. FA is a scalar derivative of DTI that demonstrates the directionality and coherence of fibre tracts, which are further dependent on microstructural parameters in a voxel, but a more favourable and stronger correlation between anisotropy of diffusion and axonal density has been discovered [3, 4].

As a result, FA has the potential to be a reliable imaging marker in neurodegenerative diseases. ROI analysis is a quantitative method for measuring FA values in GM and WM of the brain areas, but its use in clinical practice must be thoroughly validated for accurate diagnosis. Error correction and standardized ROI placement are the bare minima for consistent DTI metrics, and they should be simple. DTI's utility in comparison with common brain MRI or other advanced MRI techniques has been evaluated in studies, and its use in clinical settings will be one of the most recent trends in medical imaging shortly.

10.4.1 Significance of Inclusion of GM and WM for FA in PD

The following GM and WM regions of the brain were assessed using an ROI technique: CC, CS, pons, SN, thalamus, cerebral peduncles, cerebellar peduncles, CN and putamen. The decision to include both the GM and WM regions of the brain was formulated after a thorough review of the literature on PD in which FA values demonstrated potential as imaging markers [5–8].

10.4.2 Substantia Nigra and Early PD

The study employed ROI analysis, which revealed that FA in the SN was statistically relevant and low in the PD group, implying that the PD group had GM abnormalities, which is consistent with the global studies [9–11]. FA value in the SN was low in PD patients, implying that ruination to this area is associated with changes in early PD, which is in line with research findings reported to date [5, 12–16].

It has been proposed that brain damage causes axonal loss, which is indirectly related to changes in FA. Reduction in FA at the SN of PD patients is a result of neuronal loss. As a result, DTI is a very effective method for diagnosing early PD cases. Some studies cite the SN as a good biomarker for PD, while others found no statistically significant differences in the PD group compared to controls.

10.4.3 Putamen and Early PD

A 2017 meta-analysis focused primarily on the subcortical GM, cortical GM, WM and cerebellar territory and found noteworthy findings in many areas, including the SN, caudate, putamen, CST, olfactory cortex, CC WM and globus pallidus [6]. The results of the current study revealed significant changes in the SN, putamen, CC and cerebral peduncles. Low FA at the putamen could be used to predict PD early on. A similar study linked putamen FA changes to disease progression in PD, citing an increase in FA and involvement of brain GM [17].

According to the recent research findings, the importance of FA putamen in early PD can be characterized as low FA, but as the duration of the disease increases, FA may be higher. Iron accumulation in the SN has been noted in PD patients, where increased iron levels cause an increase in FA at the putamen. This should also be considered when interpreting the putaminal FA for the routine practice [18–20].

10.4.4 Corpus Callosum and Early PD

The current study found a considerable difference in FA between PD and control groups at the genu (CC) and body (CC). In the late stages of PD, there is a significant volume loss at the CC. However, an increased FA at the CC in the PD group compared to controls in our findings could be a classic feature of early PD cases exclusively. As a result, the exploration of elevated FA in the genu (CC) and body (CC) appears worthy of mention and can be used for predicting the disease onset in early PD cases, which is noteworthy evidence that has yet to be reviewed. As the disease progresses in PD, dementia, Lewy body appearance, PD-Plus syndromes and Alzheimer's disease become involved, which may result in a decrease in FA value as the total volume of the CC decreases [21, 22]. While distinguishing between cases of early and late PD, this trend in the CC must be carefully monitored. Anisotropy is influenced by the structural arrangement of neurons, their compact size and interneuronal space. A new occurrence of a disease that disrupts its normal structure may cause an immediate increase in FA at the CC, but as the disease condition worsens, FA values generally fall and are low.

The utility of the CC as an imaging biomarker in early PD cases is still unknown, and long-term studies are needed to determine its true significance [23, 24]. Previous research on the splenium of the CC has been found to be useful in distinguishing between patients and controls with memory disorders [25], while the current study findings found no link between FA and the splenium of the CC. In a similar study on the CC and cingulum pathways, no significant variations in FA were found between the PD and control groups [26].

Because the CC is the most important link between the cerebral hemispheres, linking degeneration of interhemispheric connections to increased FA in the CC genu may shed light on overall volume reduction in the brain matter space [26]. This significant change in FA at the CC can also be linked to decreased axonal density and fibre degeneration caused by cortical damage.

Overall, if we compare FA at the CC as a whole, the study findings are consistent with the majority of the studies conducted and reported using DTI and FA. FA values reported are either higher or lower than control group values, and this finding must be correlated with the age group and type of PD cases included, namely, early or late PD.

10.4.5 Cerebral Peduncles and Early PD

FA levels in the cerebral peduncles differed statistically between groups, with the PD group having higher FA than the control group. A limited number of clinical trials have investigated the relationship between CP and FA, and none of them have produced significant results for using CP as an imaging biomarker for the early PD [27, 28]. In the majority of the studies reported, FA of the CP was used as a reference to compare with the disease group. As a result, future research with bigger sample size is required to assess the usefulness of using the cerebral peduncle as an imaging biomarker for detecting PD.

10.4.6 Pons and Early PD

Using an independent sample "*t*-test", FA at the pons revealed a statistical difference, with high FA in the PD group than the control group. Logistic regression analysis at the pons revealed no strong association between PD and the control group. As a result, the current study findings cast doubt on the utility of pons as an imaging marker. Table 10.6 depicts a comparative summary of FA in PD based on studies reported in the literature.

Table 10.6 FA in PD at the GM and WM regions of the brain with studies reported in the literature

Study reference (PD vs. control)	Regions studied	Differences in FA (statistically significant)
Current findings	CC, CS, PO, CP, CPP, P, CN, T, SN	SN↓, P↓, CC↑, CP ↑
[29]	Ca, GP, P, SN, T	SN↓
[14]	SN, CP	SN↓
[30]	CST, SLF, CI, CC	CC↓, SLF↓
[31]	SN	Not significant
[32]	CC, CI	Not significant
[33]	T, P, SN, C, PA, RN	SN↓, T↓
[34]	AOS, OT, SN, T, CST, CI, SLF, UF, ITG, F	CST↓, SLF↓, CI↓, F↓
[35]	PG, SN, T, P, IC	SN↓,P↓, T↓
[27]	P, CPP	Not significant

AOS anterior olfactory structures, *BG* basal ganglia, *C* controls, *CA* caudate, *CI* cingulum, *CC* corpus callosum, *CS* centrum semiovale, *CST* corticospinal tract, *DN* dentate nucleus, *CP* cerebral peduncles, *CN* caudate nucleus, *EC* external capsule, *F* forceps, *GP* globus pallidus, *IC* internal capsule, *ITG* inferior temporal gyrus, *LD* longitudinal diffusivity, *CPP* cerebellar peduncles, *NA* not applicable, *NS* not significant, *P* putamen, *PA* palladium, *PO* pons, *PD* Parkinson's disease, *PG* precentral gyrus, *PMC* premotor cortex, *POC* primary olfactory cortex, *RN* red nucleus, *SCP* superior cerebellar peduncles, *SN* substantia nigra, *SLF* superior longitudinal fasciculus, *T* thalamus, *UF* uncinate fasciculus

10.5 Brain Region Involvement in Early PD

The involvement of both GM and WM regions of the brain was hypothesized in our study and found to be statistically significant. The involvement of SN has already been proven useful by numerous studies reported in the literature [14–16, 35]. The role of the CC is still unclear in early PD cases, but the current study found statistically significant data for FA in early PD compared to the controls [21, 22]. FA at the putamen was also found useful and statistically significant in PD compared to its counterpart controls and can be useful for early PD detection similar to limited studies reported in literature [18, 36]. However, the present study also included the following regions for FA calculation: caudate nucleus, thalamus, cerebellar peduncles and centrum semiovale. We were unable to find any noteworthy association in these regions for the early PD group of patients. However, the involvement of the CN and thalamus might be seen in FA in the later stage of the disease [15].

Hence, the use of DTI in early PD was found useful in both GM and WM regions of the brain.

10.5.1 Conventional MRI vs. DTI in PD

Early detection of PD allows clinicians to treat patients and improve their well-being and prognosis. Because PD manifests slowly within the brain, routine MRI scans fail to detect any microstructural changes. Routine brain MRI using fluid-attenuated inversion recovery (FLAIR) and other routine sequences can show age-related and degenerative changes, but their overall diagnostic value in PD is low. In most PD cases, structural brain MRI findings are normal, and the role of MRI imaging in PD has been strictly to rule out secondary causes.

As a result, DTI with FA values should be considered a routine method for imaging diagnosis in PD cases.

10.6 Clinical and Future Implications

According to the research findings of the current study discussed earlier in this chapter, FA values at the SN are the best imaging marker for early PD cases. The discovery at the putamen makes it an early imaging biomarker for early PD cases. The current findings also found CC and cerebral peduncles to be an important imaging biomarker for the detection and early diagnosis of PD, but they also recommend more long-term studies to confirm their value.

The SN, putamen, cerebral peduncles and CC were identified as potential imaging markers for early PD detection and differentiation between PD patients and controls. DTI revealed new information about the altered microstructure of the aforementioned brain regions in early PD, potentially improving in vivo diagnostic accuracy.

Future studies comparing physiological changes in WM and GM with pathological circumstances in PD in clinical cases will be extremely useful for interpretation. The large clinical implementation of DTI and FA, in particular, will continue to evolve as we learn and study anisotropy and diffusivity in great detail.

Future research could look into whether preclinical DTI results can be used to predict the progression of dementia and parkinsonian syndromes. The prospect of a delicate, specific MRI biomarker is clinically extremely desirable, and more research is needed to target this. Longitudinal studies on large cohorts will be especially useful because they will allow the impact of disease progression to be measured. Multimodal imaging, which combines various methods such as SN iron quantification, can improve diagnostic sensitivity and is an important research direction. Longitudinal studies may lead to techniques for identifying those at risk of cognitive dysfunction and later dementia-related PD, allowing for earlier intervention and distinguishing between early and late PD instances.

There is also a need to investigate the effects of antiparkinsonian medicines on diffusion-tensor measurements in tests. Higher field strengths of 3 T could produce clinically interesting DTI results by increasing signal sensitivity and thus image resolution.

References

1. Hughes AJ, Daniel SE, Kilford L, Lees AJ, Daniel SE. Accuracy of clinical diagnosis of idiopathic Parkinson's disease: a clinico-pathological study of 100 cases. Neurosurg Psychiatry. 1991;55(55):181–4. http://www.ncbi.nlm.nih.gov/pubmed/1564476.
2. Saeed U, Compagnone J, Aviv RI, Strafella AP, Black SE, Lang AE, et al. Imaging biomarkers in Parkinson's disease and Parkinsonian syndromes: current and emerging concepts. Transl Neurodegener. 2017;6:8.
3. Wahl M, Lauterbach-Soon B, Hattingen E, Jung P, Singer O, Volz S, et al. Human motor corpus callosum: topography, somatotopy, and link between microstructure and function. J Neurosci. 2007;27(45):12132–8. http://www.jneurosci.org/cgi/doi/10.1523/JNEUROSCI.2320-07.2007.
4. Ito M, Watanabe H, Kawai Y, Atsuta N, Tanaka F, Naganawa S, et al. Usefulness of combined fractional anisotropy and apparent diffusion coefficient values for detection of involvement in multiple system atrophy. J Neurol Neurosurg Psychiatry. 2007;78(7):722–8.
5. Cochrane CJ, Ebmeier KP. Diffusion tensor imaging in parkinsonian syndromes: a systematic review and meta-analysis. Neurology. 2013;80(9):857–64.
6. Atkinson-Clement C, Pinto S, Eusebio A, Coulon O. Diffusion tensor imaging in Parkinson's disease: review and meta-analysis. NeuroImage Clin. 2017;16:98–110.
7. Kotian RP, Prakashini K, Nair NS. A diffusion tensor imaging study to compare normative fractional anisotropy values with patients suffering from Parkinson's disease in the brain grey and white matter. Health Technol (Berl). 2020;10(5):1283–9. https://doi.org/10.1007/s12553-020-00454-1.
8. Kotian RP, Sreekumaran Nair N, Babu SM. A diffusion tensor imaging study to estimate normative fractional anisotropy values in different age groups of normal brain white matter. Int J Control Theory Appl. 2017;10(36):195–204.
9. Schwarz ST, Abaei M, Gontu V, Morgan PS, Bajaj N, Auer DP. Diffusion tensor imaging of nigral degeneration in Parkinson's disease: a region-of-interest and voxel-based study at 3 T and systematic review with meta-analysis. NeuroImage Clin. 2013;3:481–8. https://doi.org/10.1016/j.nicl.2013.10.006.
10. Melzer TR, Watts R, Macaskill MR, Pitcher TL, Livingston L, Keenan RJ, et al. White matter microstructure deteriorates across cognitive stages in Parkinson disease. Neurology. 2013;80(20):1841–9.
11. Pozorski V, Oh JM, Adluru N, Merluzzi AP, Theisen F, Okonkwo O, et al. Longitudinal white matter microstructural change in Parkinson's disease. Hum Brain Mapp. 2018;39(10):4150–61.
12. Prakash BD, Sitoh Y-Y, Tan LCS, Au WL. Asymmetrical diffusion tensor imaging indices of the rostral substantia nigra in Parkinson's disease. Parkinsonism Relat Disord. 2012;18(9):1029–33. https://linkinghub.elsevier.com/retrieve/pii/S135380201200209X.
13. Zhang Y, Wu IW, Tosun D, Foster E, Schuff N. Progression of regional microstructural degeneration in Parkinson's disease: a multicenter diffusion tensor imaging study. PLoS One. 2016;11(10):1–16.
14. Vaillancourt DE, Spraker MB, Prodoehl J, Abraham I, Corcos DM, Zhou XJ, et al. High-resolution diffusion tensor imaging in the substantia nigra of de novo Parkinson disease. Neurology. 2009;72(16):1378–84. http://www.neurology.org/cgi/doi/10.1212/01.wnl.0000340982.01727.6e.
15. Péran P, Cherubini A, Assogna F, Piras F, Quattrocchi C, Peppe A, et al. Magnetic resonance imaging markers of Parkinson's disease nigrostriatal signature. Brain. 2010;133(11):3423–33. https://academic.oup.com/brain/article-lookup/doi/10.1093/brain/awq212.
16. Chan L-L, Rumpel H, Yap K, Lee E, Loo H-V, Ho G-L, et al. Case control study of diffusion tensor imaging in Parkinson's disease. J Neurol Neurosurg Psychiatry. 2007;78(12):1383–6. http://www.ncbi.nlm.nih.gov/pubmed/17615165

17. Chan LL, Ng KM, Yeoh CS, Rumpel H, Li HH, Tan EK. Putaminal diffusivity correlates with disease progression in Parkinson's disease. Medicine (Baltimore). 2016;95(6):e2594.
18. Rulseh AM, Keller J, Tintěra J, Kožíšek M, Vymazal J. Chasing shadows: what determines DTI metrics in gray matter regions? An in vitro and in vivo study. J Magn Reson Imaging. 2013;38(5):1103–10. https://doi.org/10.1002/jmri.24065.
19. Pfefferbaum A, Adalsteinsson E, Rohlfing T, Sullivan EV. Diffusion tensor imaging of deep gray matter brain structures: effects of age and iron concentration. Neurobiol Aging. 2010;31(3):482–93. https://linkinghub.elsevier.com/retrieve/pii/S0197458008001401.
20. White ML, Zhang Y. Three-tesla diffusion tensor imaging of Meyer's loop by tractography, color-coded fractional anisotropy maps, and eigenvectors. Clin Imaging. 2010;34(6):413–7. http://www.sciencedirect.com/science/article/pii/S0899707110000021.
21. Goldman JG, Bledsoe IO, Merkitch D, Dinh V, Bernard B, Stebbins GT. Corpus callosal atrophy and associations with cognitive impairment in Parkinson disease. Neurology. 2017;88(13):1265–72. http://www.neurology.org/lookup/doi/10.1212/WNL.0000000000003764.
22. Wiltshire K, Foster S, Kaye JA, Small BJ, Camicioli R. Corpus callosum in neurodegenerative diseases: findings in Parkinson's disease. Dement Geriatr Cogn Disord. 2005;20(6):345–51. http://www.ncbi.nlm.nih.gov/pubmed/16192724.
23. Boelmans K, Christian N, Suchorska B, Kaufmann J, Ebersbach G, Heinze H, et al. Parkinsonism and related disorders diffusion tensor imaging of the corpus callosum differentiates corticobasal syndrome from Parkinson's disease q. Parkisonism Relat Disord. 2017;16(8):498–502. https://doi.org/10.1016/j.parkreldis.2010.05.006.
24. Schwarz ST, Abaei M, Gontu V, Morgan PS, Bajaj N, Auer DP. NeuroImage: clinical diffusion tensor imaging of nigral degeneration in Parkinson's disease: a region-of-interest and voxel-based study at 3T and systematic review with meta-analysis. Neuroimage Clin. 2013;3:481–8. https://doi.org/10.1016/j.nicl.2013.10.006.
25. Zhuang L, Wen W, Zhu W, Trollor J, Kochan N, Crawford J, et al. White matter integrity in mild cognitive impairment: a tract-based spatial statistics study. Neuroimage. 2010;53(1):16–25. https://doi.org/10.1016/j.neuroimage.2010.05.068.
26. Concha L, Bouchard T, Wiltshire K, Concha L, Gee M, Bouchard T. Corpus callosum and cingulum tractography in Parkinson's disease. Can J Neurol Sci. 2010;37(5):595–600.
27. Meijer FJA, Van RA, Tuladhar AM. Conventional 3T brain MRI and diffusion tensor imaging in the diagnostic workup of early stage parkinsonism. Neuroradiology. 2015;57(7):655–69. https://doi.org/10.1007/s00234-015-1515-7.
28. Meijer FJA, Bloem BR, Mahlknecht P, Seppi K, Goraj B. Update on diffusion MRI in Parkinson's disease and atypical parkinsonism. J Neurol Sci. 2013;332(1–2):21–9. https://doi.org/10.1016/j.jns.2013.06.032.
29. Chan L, Rumpel H, Yap K, Lee E, Loo H, Ho G, et al. disease. 2007;1383–6.
30. Gattellaro G, Minati L, Grisoli M, Mariani C, Carella F, Osio M, et al. White matter involvement in idiopathic Parkinson disease: a diffusion tensor imaging study. AJNR Am J Neuroradiol. 2009;30(6):1222–6.
31. Menke RA, Scholz J, Miller KL, Deoni S, Jbabdi S, Matthews PM, et al. MRI characteristics of the substantia nigra in Parkinson's disease: a combined quantitative T1 and DTI study. Neuroimage. 2009;47(2):435–41. https://linkinghub.elsevier.com/retrieve/pii/S1053811909004935.
32. Wiltshire K, Concha L, Gee M, Bouchard T, Beaulieu C, Camicioli R. Corpus callosum and cingulum tractography in Parkinson's disease. Can J Neurol Sci. 2010;37(5):595–600. http://www.ncbi.nlm.nih.gov/pubmed/21059504.
33. Péran P, Cherubini A, Assogna F, Piras F, Quattrocchi C, Peppe A, et al. Magnetic resonance imaging markers of Parkinson's disease nigrostriatal signature. Brain. 2010;133(11):3423–33. http://www.ncbi.nlm.nih.gov/pubmed/20736190
34. Chen N-K, Chou Y, Sundman M, Hickey P, Kasoff WS, Bernstein A, et al. Alteration of diffusion-tensor MRI measures in brain regions involved in early stages of Parkinson's disease. Brain Connect. 2018;8(6):343–9. http://www.liebertpub.com/doi/10.1089/brain.2017.0558.

35. Zhan W, Kang GA, Glass GA, Zhang Y, Shirley C, Millin R, et al. Regional alterations of brain microstructure in Parkinson's disease using diffusion tensor imaging. Mov Disord. 2012;27(1):90–7.
36. Pfefferbaum A, Adalsteinsson E, Rohlfing T, Sullivan EV. Diffusion tensor imaging of deep gray matter brain structures: effects of age and iron concentration. Neurobiol Aging. 2010;31(3):482–93. http://www.pubmedcentral.nih.gov/articlerender.fcgi?artid=2815127&tool=pmcentrez&rendertype=abstract.

Glossary

ADC Apparent diffusion coefficient
AOS Anterior olfactory structures
B_0 Magnetic field strength
BG Basal ganglia
b-Value **b value** measures the degree of diffusion-weighting applied, thereby indicating the amplitude (G), time of applied gradients (δ) and duration between the paired gradients (Δ) and is calculated as: $b = \gamma^2 G^2 \delta^2(\Delta - \delta/3)$.
C Controls
CA Caudate
CC Corpus callosum
CG Cingulum
CI Cingulum
CP Cerebral peduncles
CS Centrum semiovale
CSF Cerebrospinal fluid
CST Corticospinal tract
CT Computed tomography
DN Dentate nucleus
DTI Diffusion tensor imaging
DWI Diffusion-weighted imaging
EC External capsule
EPI Echo planar imaging
F Forceps
FA Fractional anisotropy
FID Free induction decay
Flip angle Flip angle is an MRI phenomenon by which the axis of the hydrogen proton shifts from its longitudinal plane (static magnetic field B_0) Z axis to its transverse plane XY axis by excitation with the help of radiofrequency (RF) pulses.
Fourier transform The Fourier transform is a mathematical technique that allows an MR signal to be decomposed into a sum of sine waves of different frequencies, phases and amplitudes.

R. P. Kotian, P. Koteshwar, *Diffusion Tensor Imaging and Fractional Anisotropy*,
https://doi.org/10.1007/978-981-19-5001-8

FOV Field of view

Functional MRI Measures brain activity by detecting changes associated with blood flow.

GM Grey matter

GP Globus pallidus

Gradient Gradients are loops of wire or thin conductive sheets on a cylindrical shell lying just inside the bore of an MR scanner. When current is passed through these coils, a secondary magnetic field is created.

Gradient echo/GE **Gradient echo sequences (GRE)** are an alternative technique to spin-echo sequences, differing from it in two principal points: (a) The utilization of gradient fields to generate transverse magnetization. (b) Flip angles of less than 90°

IC Internal capsule

IPD Idiopathic Parkinson's disease

ITG Inferior temporal gyrus

LD Longitudinal diffusivity

MCP Middle cerebral peduncles

MMSE Mini-Mental State Examination

MRI Magnetic resonance imaging

MSA Multiple system atrophy

NA Not applicable

NMV Net magnetization vector

NS Not significant

Parallel imaging techniques Parallel imaging is a widely used technique where the known placement and sensitivities of receiver coils are used to assist spatial localization of MR signal.Allows reduction in number of phase encode steps and hence imaging time.

PD Parkinson's disease

PD W Proton density-weighted image

PET Positron emission tomography

PG Precentral gyrus

PMC Premotor cortex

POC Primary olfactory cortex

Precession Spin wobble (or precess) about the axis of magnetic field.

PSP Progressive supranuclear palsy

RF Radio frequency

RN Red nucleus

ROI Region of interest

SCP Superior cerebral peduncles

SLF Superior longitudinal fasciculus

SN Substantia nigra

SPECT Single photon emission-computed tomography

Spin echo/SE Spin echo is pulse sequence generated by two successive RF pulses, typically a 90–180°pair.

SS Single shot

T1W **T1-weighted image** (also referred to as **T1W** or the "spin-lattice" relaxation time) is one of the basic pulse sequences in MRI and demonstrates differences in the T1 relaxation times of tissues.

T2W **T2-weighted image** (**T2W**) is one of the basic pulse sequences on MRI. The sequence weighting highlights differences on the T2 relaxation times of tissues.

T Tesla

TE Echo time

Th Thalamus

TR Repetition time

UF Uncinate fasciculus

UPDRS Unified Parkinson's Disease Rating Scale

WM White matter

GPSR Compliance

The European Union's (EU) General Product Safety Regulation (GPSR) is a set of rules that requires consumer products to be safe and our obligations to ensure this.

If you have any concerns about our products, you can contact us on ProductSafety@springernature.com

In case Publisher is established outside the EU, the EU authorized representative is:

Springer Nature Customer Service Center GmbH
Europaplatz 3
69115 Heidelberg, Germany

Batch number: 10370708

Printed by Printforce, the Netherlands